Daily Habit Tracker

Small Steps Lead To Big Results

Month ___________________

Year ___________________

Goal

Day								
1								
2								
3								
4								
5								
6								
7								

Daily Habit Tracker
Small Steps Lead To Big Results

Month _____________

Year _____________

Goal

Day

1

2

3

4

5

6

7

This is a weekly habit tracker to keep track of even the smallest of habits. Whether it's just reading one page of a book or doing one pushup or putting away the laundry. Small steps lead to big results over time.

So whatever your goal is and whatever habit you want to start then use this book as a guide to keep you on track.

Best of luck to you!!

Daily Habit Tracker

Small Steps Lead To Big Results

Month ___________________

Year ___________________

Goal

Day														
1														
2														
3														
4														
5														
6														
7														

Daily Habit Tracker

Small Steps Lead To Big Results

Month __________

Year __________

Goal

Day													
1													
2													
3													
4													
5													
6													
7													

Daily Habit Tracker

Small Steps Lead To Big Results

Month

Year

Goal

Day															
1															
2															
3															
4															
5															
6															
7															

Daily Habit Tracker

Small Steps Lead To Big Results

Month________________

Year________________

Goal

Day															
1															
2															
3															
4															
5															
6															
7															

Daily Habit Tracker

Small Steps Lead To Big Results

Month_______________

Year_______________

Goal

Day														
1														
2														
3														
4														
5														
6														
7														

Daily Habit Tracker

Small Steps Lead To Big Results

Month ________________

Year ________________

Goal

Day														
1														
2														
3														
4														
5														
6														
7														

Daily Habit Tracker

Small Steps Lead To Big Results

Month

Year

Goal

Day

1

2

3

4

5

6

7

Daily Habit Tracker

Small Steps Lead To Big Results

Month _______________

Year _______________

Goal

Day														
1														
2														
3														
4														
5														
6														
7														

Daily Habit Tracker

Small Steps Lead To Big Results

Month ___________

Year ___________

Goal

Day															
1															
2															
3															
4															
5															
6															
7															

Daily Habit Tracker

Small Steps Lead To Big Results

Month_____________

Year_____________

Goal

Day															
1															
2															
3															
4															
5															
6															
7															

Daily Habit Tracker

Small Steps Lead To Big Results

Month ___________

Year ___________

Goal

Day														
1														
2														
3														
4														
5														
6														
7														

Daily Habit Tracker

Small Steps Lead To Big Results

Month_______________

Year_______________

Goal

Day														
1														
2														
3														
4														
5														
6														
7														

Daily Habit Tracker

Small Steps Lead To Big Results

Month_______________

Year_______________

Goal

Day															
1															
2															
3															
4															
5															
6															
7															

Daily Habit Tracker
Small Steps Lead To Big Results

Month ___________

Year ___________

Goal

Day														
1														
2														
3														
4														
5														
6														
7														

Daily Habit Tracker

Small Steps Lead To Big Results

Month _______________

Year _______________

Goal

Day															
1															
2															
3															
4															
5															
6															
7															

Daily Habit Tracker

Small Steps Lead To Big Results

Month _______________

Year _______________

Goal

Day															
1															
2															
3															
4															
5															
6															
7															

Daily Habit Tracker

Small Steps Lead To Big Results

Month ______________

Year ______________

Goal

Day															
1															
2															
3															
4															
5															
6															
7															

Daily Habit Tracker

Small Steps Lead To Big Results

Month_______________

Year_______________

Goal

Day															
1															
2															
3															
4															
5															
6															
7															

Daily Habit Tracker

Small Steps Lead To Big Results

Month

Year

Goal

Day														
1														
2														
3														
4														
5														
6														
7														

Daily Habit Tracker

Small Steps Lead To Big Results

Month

Year

Goal

Day

1

2

3

4

5

6

7

Daily Habit Tracker

Small Steps Lead To Big Results

Month _______________

Year _______________

Goal

Day
1
2
3
4
5
6
7

Daily Habit Tracker
Small Steps Lead To Big Results

Month_______________

Year_______________

Goal

Day															
1															
2															
3															
4															
5															
6															
7															

Daily Habit Tracker

Small Steps Lead To Big Results

Month _______________

Year _______________

Goal

Day															
1															
2															
3															
4															
5															
6															
7															

Daily Habit Tracker

Small Steps Lead To Big Results

Month ___________

Year ___________

Goal

Day														
1														
2														
3														
4														
5														
6														
7														

Daily Habit Tracker

Small Steps Lead To Big Results

Month_______________

Year_______________

Goal

Day														
1														
2														
3														
4														
5														
6														
7														

Daily Habit Tracker

Small Steps Lead To Big Results

Month________________

Year________________

Goal

Day															
1															
2															
3															
4															
5															
6															
7															

Daily Habit Tracker

Small Steps Lead To Big Results

Month ___________

Year ___________

Goal

Day														
1														
2														
3														
4														
5														
6														
7														

Daily Habit Tracker

Small Steps Lead To Big Results

Month _______________

Year _______________

Goal

Day														
1														
2														
3														
4														
5														
6														
7														

Daily Habit Tracker

Small Steps Lead To Big Results

Month

Year

Goal

Day

1

2

3

4

5

6

7

Daily Habit Tracker

Small Steps Lead To Big Results

Month_______________

Year_______________

Goal

Day													
1													
2													
3													
4													
5													
6													
7													

Daily Habit Tracker

Small Steps Lead To Big Results

Month

Year

Goal

Day														
1														
2														
3														
4														
5														
6														
7														

Daily Habit Tracker

Small Steps Lead To Big Results

Month _______________

Year _______________

Goal

Day															
1															
2															
3															
4															
5															
6															
7															

Daily Habit Tracker

Small Steps Lead To Big Results

Month ______________

Year ______________

Goal

Day															
1															
2															
3															
4															
5															
6															
7															

Daily Habit Tracker

Small Steps Lead To Big Results

Month_______________

Year_______________

Goal

Day															
1															
2															
3															
4															
5															
6															
7															

Daily Habit Tracker

Small Steps Lead To Big Results

Month ___________

Year ___________

Goal

Day															
1															
2															
3															
4															
5															
6															
7															

Daily Habit Tracker

Small Steps Lead To Big Results

Month _______________

Year _______________

Goal

Day														
1														
2														
3														
4														
5														
6														
7														

Daily Habit Tracker

Small Steps Lead To Big Results

Month_______________

Year_______________

Goal

Day														
1														
2														
3														
4														
5														
6														
7														

Daily Habit Tracker

Small Steps Lead To Big Results

Month_______________

Year_______________

Goal

Day														
1														
2														
3														
4														
5														
6														
7														

Daily Habit Tracker

Small Steps Lead To Big Results

Month __________

Year __________

Goal

Day															
1															
2															
3															
4															
5															
6															
7															

Daily Habit Tracker

Small Steps Lead To Big Results

Month_____________

Year_____________

Goal

Day															
1															
2															
3															
4															
5															
6															
7															

Daily Habit Tracker

Small Steps Lead To Big Results

Month________________

Year________________

Goal

Day														
1														
2														
3														
4														
5														
6														
7														

Daily Habit Tracker

Small Steps Lead To Big Results

Month

Year

Goal

Day														
1														
2														
3														
4														
5														
6														
7														

Daily Habit Tracker

Small Steps Lead To Big Results

Month_______________

Year_______________

Goal

Day													
1													
2													
3													
4													
5													
6													
7													

Daily Habit Tracker

Small Steps Lead To Big Results

Month

Year

Goal

Day														
1														
2														
3														
4														
5														
6														
7														

Daily Habit Tracker

Small Steps Lead To Big Results

Month

Year

Goal

Day														
1														
2														
3														
4														
5														
6														
7														

Daily Habit Tracker

Small Steps Lead To Big Results

Month

Year

Goal

Day															
1															
2															
3															
4															
5															
6															
7															

Daily Habit Tracker

Small Steps Lead To Big Results

Month_____________

Year_____________

Goal

Day														
1														
2														
3														
4														
5														
6														
7														

Daily Habit Tracker

Small Steps Lead To Big Results

Month ___________

Year ___________

Goal

Day															
1															
2															
3															
4															
5															
6															
7															

Daily Habit Tracker

Small Steps Lead To Big Results

Month__________

Year__________

Goal

Day													
1													
2													
3													
4													
5													
6													
7													

Daily Habit Tracker

Small Steps Lead To Big Results

Month__________

Year__________

Goal

Day
1
2
3
4
5
6
7

Daily Habit Tracker
Small Steps Lead To Big Results

Month _______________

Year _______________

Goal

Day														
1														
2														
3														
4														
5														
6														
7														

Daily Habit Tracker
Small Steps Lead To Big Results

Month ________

Year ________

Goal

Day															
1															
2															
3															
4															
5															
6															
7															

Daily Habit Tracker

Small Steps Lead To Big Results

Month

Year

Goal

Day													
1													
2													
3													
4													
5													
6													
7													

Daily Habit Tracker

Small Steps Lead To Big Results

Month ___________

Year ___________

Goal

Day															
1															
2															
3															
4															
5															
6															
7															

Daily Habit Tracker

Small Steps Lead To Big Results

Month _______________

Year _______________

Goal

Day															
1															
2															
3															
4															
5															
6															
7															

Daily Habit Tracker

Small Steps Lead To Big Results

Month ___________

Year ___________

Goal

Day															
1															
2															
3															
4															
5															
6															
7															

Daily Habit Tracker

Small Steps Lead To Big Results

Month __________

Year __________

Goal

Day																
1																
2																
3																
4																
5																
6																
7																

Daily Habit Tracker

Small Steps Lead To Big Results

Month _______________

Year _______________

Goal

Day													
1													
2													
3													
4													
5													
6													
7													

Daily Habit Tracker

Small Steps Lead To Big Results

Month ________________

Year ________________

Goal

Day															
1															
2															
3															
4															
5															
6															
7															

Daily Habit Tracker

Small Steps Lead To Big Results

Month_______________

Year_______________

Goal

Day															
1															
2															
3															
4															
5															
6															
7															

Daily Habit Tracker

Small Steps Lead To Big Results

Month_____________

Year_____________

Goal

Day														
1														
2														
3														
4														
5														
6														
7														

Daily Habit Tracker
Small Steps Lead To Big Results

Month

Year

Goal

Day														
1														
2														
3														
4														
5														
6														
7														

Daily Habit Tracker

Small Steps Lead To Big Results

Month ___________

Year ___________

Goal

Day														
1														
2														
3														
4														
5														
6														
7														

Daily Habit Tracker

Small Steps Lead To Big Results

Month_______________

Year_______________

Goal

Day															
1															
2															
3															
4															
5															
6															
7															

Daily Habit Tracker

Small Steps Lead To Big Results

Goal

Month ____________

Year ____________

Day															
1															
2															
3															
4															
5															
6															
7															

Daily Habit Tracker

Small Steps Lead To Big Results

Month

Year

Goal

Day														
1														
2														
3														
4														
5														
6														
7														

Daily Habit Tracker

Small Steps Lead To Big Results

Month__________

Year__________

Goal

Day															
1															
2															
3															
4															
5															
6															
7															

Daily Habit Tracker

Small Steps Lead To Big Results

Month_______________

Year_______________

Goal

Day															
1															
2															
3															
4															
5															
6															
7															

Daily Habit Tracker

Small Steps Lead To Big Results

Month ___________

Year ___________

Goal														
Day 1														
2														
3														
4														
5														
6														
7														

Daily Habit Tracker

Small Steps Lead To Big Results

Month_______________

Year_______________

Goal

Day															
1															
2															
3															
4															
5															
6															
7															

Daily Habit Tracker

Small Steps Lead To Big Results

Month _____________

Year _____________

Goal

Day														
1														
2														
3														
4														
5														
6														
7														

Daily Habit Tracker

Small Steps Lead To Big Results

Month_______________

Year_______________

Goal

Day

1

2

3

4

5

6

7

Daily Habit Tracker

Small Steps Lead To Big Results

Month __________

Year __________

Goal

Day														
1														
2														
3														
4														
5														
6														
7														

Daily Habit Tracker

Small Steps Lead To Big Results

Month _______________

Year _______________

Goal

Day															
1															
2															
3															
4															
5															
6															
7															

Daily Habit Tracker

Small Steps Lead To Big Results

Month

Year

Goal

Day															
1															
2															
3															
4															
5															
6															
7															

Daily Habit Tracker

Small Steps Lead To Big Results

Month_______________

Year_______________

Goal

Day																
1																
2																
3																
4																
5																
6																
7																

Daily Habit Tracker

Small Steps Lead To Big Results

Month ______________

Year ______________

Goal

Day														
1														
2														
3														
4														
5														
6														
7														

Daily Habit Tracker

Small Steps Lead To Big Results

Month________________

Year________________

Goal

Day															
1															
2															
3															
4															
5															
6															
7															

Daily Habit Tracker

Small Steps Lead To Big Results

Month _______________

Year _______________

Goal

Day														
1														
2														
3														
4														
5														
6														
7														

Daily Habit Tracker

Small Steps Lead To Big Results

Month

Year

Goal

Day															
1															
2															
3															
4															
5															
6															
7															

Daily Habit Tracker

Small Steps Lead To Big Results

Month______________

Year______________

Goal

Day

1

2

3

4

5

6

7

Daily Habit Tracker

Small Steps Lead To Big Results

Month_______________

Year_______________

Goal

Day														
1														
2														
3														
4														
5														
6														
7														

Daily Habit Tracker
Small Steps Lead To Big Results

Month ________________

Year ________________

Goal

Day														
1														
2														
3														
4														
5														
6														
7														

Daily Habit Tracker

Small Steps Lead To Big Results

Month_______________

Year_______________

Goal

Day															
1															
2															
3															
4															
5															
6															
7															

Daily Habit Tracker

Small Steps Lead To Big Results

Month_______________

Year_______________

Goal

Day															
1															
2															
3															
4															
5															
6															
7															

Daily Habit Tracker

Small Steps Lead To Big Results

Month ___________

Year ___________

Goal

Day															
1															
2															
3															
4															
5															
6															
7															

Daily Habit Tracker

Small Steps Lead To Big Results

Month _______________

Year _______________

Goal

Day															
1															
2															
3															
4															
5															
6															
7															

Daily Habit Tracker

Small Steps Lead To Big Results

Goal

Month ________________

Year ________________

Day														
1														
2														
3														
4														
5														
6														
7														

Daily Habit Tracker

Small Steps Lead To Big Results

Month _______________

Year _______________

Goal

Day														
1														
2														
3														
4														
5														
6														
7														

Daily Habit Tracker
Small Steps Lead To Big Results

Month ___________

Year ___________

Goal

Day															
1															
2															
3															
4															
5															
6															
7															

Daily Habit Tracker
Small Steps Lead To Big Results

Month_______________

Year_______________

Goal

Day															
1															
2															
3															
4															
5															
6															
7															

Daily Habit Tracker

Small Steps Lead To Big Results

Month

Year

Goal

Day														
1														
2														
3														
4														
5														
6														
7														

Daily Habit Tracker

Small Steps Lead To Big Results

Month ________________

Year ________________

Goal

Day														
1														
2														
3														
4														
5														
6														
7														

Daily Habit Tracker
Small Steps Lead To Big Results

Month _______________

Year _______________

Goal

Day														
1														
2														
3														
4														
5														
6														
7														

Daily Habit Tracker

Small Steps Lead To Big Results

Month ______________

Year ______________

Goal

Day															
1															
2															
3															
4															
5															
6															
7															

Daily Habit Tracker

Small Steps Lead To Big Results

Month_______________

Year_______________

Goal

Day													
1													
2													
3													
4													
5													
6													
7													

Daily Habit Tracker

Small Steps Lead To Big Results

Month_______________

Year_______________

Goal

Day														
1														
2														
3														
4														
5														
6														
7														

Daily Habit Tracker

Small Steps Lead To Big Results

Month__________

Year__________

Goal

Day															
1															
2															
3															
4															
5															
6															
7															

Daily Habit Tracker

Small Steps Lead To Big Results

Month ____________

Year ____________

Goal

Day															
1															
2															
3															
4															
5															
6															
7															

Daily Habit Tracker

Small Steps Lead To Big Results

Month_____________

Year_____________

Goal

Day														
1														
2														
3														
4														
5														
6														
7														

Daily Habit Tracker

Small Steps Lead To Big Results

Month __________

Year __________

Goal

Day																
1																
2																
3																
4																
5																
6																
7																

Daily Habit Tracker

Small Steps Lead To Big Results

Month __________

Year __________

Goal

Day														
1														
2														
3														
4														
5														
6														
7														

Daily Habit Tracker

Small Steps Lead To Big Results

Month_____________

Year_____________

Goal

Day														
1														
2														
3														
4														
5														
6														
7														

Daily Habit Tracker
Small Steps Lead To Big Results

Month _______________

Year _______________

Goal

Day															
1															
2															
3															
4															
5															
6															
7															

Daily Habit Tracker

Small Steps Lead To Big Results

Month_______________

Year_______________

Goal

Day															
1															
2															
3															
4															
5															
6															
7															

Daily Habit Tracker
Small Steps Lead To Big Results

Month_____________

Year_____________

Goal

Day															
1															
2															
3															
4															
5															
6															
7															

Daily Habit Tracker

Small Steps Lead To Big Results

Month ______________

Year ______________

Goal

Day														
1														
2														
3														
4														
5														
6														
7														

Daily Habit Tracker

Small Steps Lead To Big Results

Month _______________

Year _______________

Goal

Day															
1															
2															
3															
4															
5															
6															
7															

Daily Habit Tracker

Small Steps Lead To Big Results

Month _______________

Year _______________

Goal														
Day 1														
2														
3														
4														
5														
6														
7														

Daily Habit Tracker

Small Steps Lead To Big Results

Month_______________

Year_______________

Goal

Day														
1														
2														
3														
4														
5														
6														
7														

Daily Habit Tracker

Small Steps Lead To Big Results

Month____________________

Year____________________

Goal

Day													
1													
2													
3													
4													
5													
6													
7													

Daily Habit Tracker

Small Steps Lead To Big Results

Month ______________

Year ______________

Goal

Day														
1														
2														
3														
4														
5														
6														
7														

Daily Habit Tracker

Small Steps Lead To Big Results

Month ___________

Year ___________

Goal

Day															
1															
2															
3															
4															
5															
6															
7															

Daily Habit Tracker

Small Steps Lead To Big Results

Month ______________

Year ______________

Goal

Day	Goal															
1																
2																
3																
4																
5																
6																
7																

Daily Habit Tracker

Small Steps Lead To Big Results

Month ___________

Year ___________

Goal

Day														
1														
2														
3														
4														
5														
6														
7														

Daily Habit Tracker

Small Steps Lead To Big Results

Month

Year

Goal

Day
1
2
3
4
5
6
7

Daily Habit Tracker

Small Steps Lead To Big Results

Month _______________

Year _______________

Goal

Day														
1														
2														
3														
4														
5														
6														
7														

Daily Habit Tracker

Small Steps Lead To Big Results

Month ________________

Year ________________

Goal

Day														
1														
2														
3														
4														
5														
6														
7														

Daily Habit Tracker
Small Steps Lead To Big Results

Goal

Month __________

Year __________

Day														
1														
2														
3														
4														
5														
6														
7														

Daily Habit Tracker

Small Steps Lead To Big Results

Month________________

Year________________

Goal

Day															
1															
2															
3															
4															
5															
6															
7															

Daily Habit Tracker

Small Steps Lead To Big Results

Month _______________

Year _______________

Goal

Day														
1														
2														
3														
4														
5														
6														
7														

Daily Habit Tracker
Small Steps Lead To Big Results

Month_____________

Year_____________

Goal

Day															
1															
2															
3															
4															
5															
6															
7															

Daily Habit Tracker

Small Steps Lead To Big Results

Month ________________

Year ________________

Goal

Day														
1														
2														
3														
4														
5														
6														
7														

Daily Habit Tracker
Small Steps Lead To Big Results

Month__________

Year__________

Goal

Day														
1														
2														
3														
4														
5														
6														
7														

Daily Habit Tracker

Small Steps Lead To Big Results

Month

Year

Goal

Day														
1														
2														
3														
4														
5														
6														
7														

Daily Habit Tracker

Small Steps Lead To Big Results

Month_______________

Year_______________

Goal

Day															
1															
2															
3															
4															
5															
6															
7															

Daily Habit Tracker

Small Steps Lead To Big Results

Month________________

Year________________

Goal

Day															
1															
2															
3															
4															
5															
6															
7															

Daily Habit Tracker
Small Steps Lead To Big Results

Month_______________

Year_______________

Goal

Day															
1															
2															
3															
4															
5															
6															
7															

Daily Habit Tracker

Small Steps Lead To Big Results

Month________________

Year________________

Goal

Day														
1														
2														
3														
4														
5														
6														
7														

Daily Habit Tracker

Small Steps Lead To Big Results

Month

Year

Goal

Day														
1														
2														
3														
4														
5														
6														
7														

Daily Habit Tracker

Small Steps Lead To Big Results

Month ______________

Year ______________

Goal

Day														
1														
2														
3														
4														
5														
6														
7														

Daily Habit Tracker

Small Steps Lead To Big Results

Month________________

Year________________

Goal

Day															
1															
2															
3															
4															
5															
6															
7															

Daily Habit Tracker

Small Steps Lead To Big Results

Month ______________

Year ______________

Goal

Day															
1															
2															
3															
4															
5															
6															
7															

Daily Habit Tracker

Small Steps Lead To Big Results

Month ________________

Year ________________

Goal

Day															
1															
2															
3															
4															
5															
6															
7															

Daily Habit Tracker
Small Steps Lead To Big Results

Month ___________

Year ___________

Goal

Day																
1																
2																
3																
4																
5																
6																
7																

Daily Habit Tracker

Small Steps Lead To Big Results

Month _______________

Year _______________

Goal

Day															
1															
2															
3															
4															
5															
6															
7															

Daily Habit Tracker

Small Steps Lead To Big Results

Month________________

Year________________

Goal

Day															
1															
2															
3															
4															
5															
6															
7															

Daily Habit Tracker

Small Steps Lead To Big Results

Month_______________

Year_______________

Goal

Day															
1															
2															
3															
4															
5															
6															
7															

Daily Habit Tracker

Small Steps Lead To Big Results

Month ________

Year ________

Goal

Day															
1															
2															
3															
4															
5															
6															
7															

Daily Habit Tracker

Small Steps Lead To Big Results

Month __________

Year __________

Goal

Day															
1															
2															
3															
4															
5															
6															
7															

Daily Habit Tracker

Small Steps Lead To Big Results

Month________________

Year________________

Goal

Day														
1														
2														
3														
4														
5														
6														
7														

Daily Habit Tracker

Small Steps Lead To Big Results

Month________________

Year________________

Goal

Day														
1														
2														
3														
4														
5														
6														
7														

Daily Habit Tracker

Small Steps Lead To Big Results

Month ___________

Year ___________

Goal

Day														
1														
2														
3														
4														
5														
6														
7														

Daily Habit Tracker

Small Steps Lead To Big Results

Month _______________

Year _______________

Goal

Day														
1														
2														
3														
4														
5														
6														
7														

Daily Habit Tracker

Small Steps Lead To Big Results

Goal

Month _______________

Year _______________

Day														
1														
2														
3														
4														
5														
6														
7														

Daily Habit Tracker

Small Steps Lead To Big Results

Month_______________

Year_______________

Goal

Day														
1														
2														
3														
4														
5														
6														
7														

Daily Habit Tracker

Small Steps Lead To Big Results

Month_______________

Year_______________

Goal

Day
1
2
3
4
5
6
7

Daily Habit Tracker

Small Steps Lead To Big Results

Month

Year

Goal

Day															
1															
2															
3															
4															
5															
6															
7															

Daily Habit Tracker

Small Steps Lead To Big Results

Month ___________

Year ___________

Goal

Day													
1													
2													
3													
4													
5													
6													
7													

Daily Habit Tracker

Small Steps Lead To Big Results

Month_______________

Year_______________

Goal

Day														
1														
2														
3														
4														
5														
6														
7														

Daily Habit Tracker

Small Steps Lead To Big Results

Month

Year

Goal

Day														
1														
2														
3														
4														
5														
6														
7														

Daily Habit Tracker

Small Steps Lead To Big Results

Month

Year

Goal

Day														
1														
2														
3														
4														
5														
6														
7														

Daily Habit Tracker

Small Steps Lead To Big Results

Month____________

Year____________

Goal

Day															
1															
2															
3															
4															
5															
6															
7															

Daily Habit Tracker

Small Steps Lead To Big Results

Month ______________

Year ______________

Goal

Day														
1														
2														
3														
4														
5														
6														
7														

Daily Habit Tracker

Small Steps Lead To Big Results

Month_____________

Year_____________

Goal															
Day 1															
2															
3															
4															
5															
6															
7															

Daily Habit Tracker

Small Steps Lead To Big Results

Month ___________

Year ___________

Goal

Day															
1															
2															
3															
4															
5															
6															
7															

Daily Habit Tracker

Small Steps Lead To Big Results

Month ___________

Year ___________

Goal

Day														
1														
2														
3														
4														
5														
6														
7														

Daily Habit Tracker

Small Steps Lead To Big Results

Month________________

Year________________

Goal

Day															
1															
2															
3															
4															
5															
6															
7															

Daily Habit Tracker

Small Steps Lead To Big Results

Month_______________

Year_______________

Goal

Day														
1														
2														
3														
4														
5														
6														
7														

Daily Habit Tracker

Small Steps Lead To Big Results

Month ________________

Year ________________

Goal

Day														
1														
2														
3														
4														
5														
6														
7														

Daily Habit Tracker

Small Steps Lead To Big Results

Month_______________

Year_______________

Goal

Day														
1														
2														
3														
4														
5														
6														
7														

Daily Habit Tracker

Small Steps Lead To Big Results

Month______________

Year______________

Goal

Day													
1													
2													
3													
4													
5													
6													
7													

Daily Habit Tracker

Small Steps Lead To Big Results

Goal

Month __________

Year __________

Day														
1														
2														
3														
4														
5														
6														
7														

Daily Habit Tracker

Small Steps Lead To Big Results

Month_______________

Year_______________

Goal

Day														
1														
2														
3														
4														
5														
6														
7														

Daily Habit Tracker

Small Steps Lead To Big Results

Month________________

Year________________

Goal

Day															
1															
2															
3															
4															
5															
6															
7															

Daily Habit Tracker

Small Steps Lead To Big Results

Month ______________

Year ______________

Goal

Day															
1															
2															
3															
4															
5															
6															
7															

Daily Habit Tracker
Small Steps Lead To Big Results

Month

Year

Goal

Day															
1															
2															
3															
4															
5															
6															
7															

Daily Habit Tracker

Small Steps Lead To Big Results

Month________

Year________

Goal

Day													
1													
2													
3													
4													
5													
6													
7													

Daily Habit Tracker

Small Steps Lead To Big Results

Month

Year

Goal

Day															
1															
2															
3															
4															
5															
6															
7															

Daily Habit Tracker

Small Steps Lead To Big Results

Month_______________

Year_______________

Goal

Day															
1															
2															
3															
4															
5															
6															
7															

Daily Habit Tracker

Small Steps Lead To Big Results

Month ______________

Year ______________

Goal

Day													
1													
2													
3													
4													
5													
6													
7													

Daily Habit Tracker

Small Steps Lead To Big Results

Month ___________

Year ___________

Goal

Day

1

2

3

4

5

6

7

Daily Habit Tracker

Small Steps Lead To Big Results

Month _______________

Year _______________

Goal

Day														
1														
2														
3														
4														
5														
6														
7														

Daily Habit Tracker

Small Steps Lead To Big Results

Month_______________

Year_______________

Goal

Day														
1														
2														
3														
4														
5														
6														
7														

Daily Habit Tracker

Small Steps Lead To Big Results

Month ______________

Year ______________

Goal

Day															
1															
2															
3															
4															
5															
6															
7															

Daily Habit Tracker

Small Steps Lead To Big Results

Month ________________

Year ________________

Goal

Day														
1														
2														
3														
4														
5														
6														
7														

Daily Habit Tracker

Small Steps Lead To Big Results

Month ___________

Year ___________

Goal

Day														
1														
2														
3														
4														
5														
6														
7														

Daily Habit Tracker

Small Steps Lead To Big Results

Month_______________

Year_______________

Goal

Day															
1															
2															
3															
4															
5															
6															
7															

Daily Habit Tracker

Small Steps Lead To Big Results

Month ___________

Year ___________

Goal

Day																
1																
2																
3																
4																
5																
6																
7																

Daily Habit Tracker

Small Steps Lead To Big Results

Month ___________

Year ___________

Goal

Day														
1														
2														
3														
4														
5														
6														
7														

Daily Habit Tracker
Small Steps Lead To Big Results

Month ___________

Year ___________

Goal

Day															
1															
2															
3															
4															
5															
6															
7															

Daily Habit Tracker

Small Steps Lead To Big Results

Month_____________

Year_____________

Goal

Day															
1															
2															
3															
4															
5															
6															
7															

Daily Habit Tracker

Small Steps Lead To Big Results

Month_____________

Year_____________

Goal

Day															
1															
2															
3															
4															
5															
6															
7															

Daily Habit Tracker
Small Steps Lead To Big Results

Month ______________

Year ______________

Goal

Day															
1															
2															
3															
4															
5															
6															
7															

Daily Habit Tracker

Small Steps Lead To Big Results

Month_______________

Year_______________

Goal

Day															
1															
2															
3															
4															
5															
6															
7															

Daily Habit Tracker

Small Steps Lead To Big Results

Month ______________

Year ______________

Goal

Day														
1														
2														
3														
4														
5														
6														
7														

Daily Habit Tracker

Small Steps Lead To Big Results

Month ___________

Year ___________

Goal

Day														
1														
2														
3														
4														
5														
6														
7														

Daily Habit Tracker

Small Steps Lead To Big Results

Month______________

Year______________

Goal

Day															
1															
2															
3															
4															
5															
6															
7															

Daily Habit Tracker

Small Steps Lead To Big Results

Month ___________

Year ___________

Goal

Day														
1														
2														
3														
4														
5														
6														
7														

Daily Habit Tracker

Small Steps Lead To Big Results

Month_______________

Year_______________

Goal

Day													
1													
2													
3													
4													
5													
6													
7													

Daily Habit Tracker

Small Steps Lead To Big Results

Month_____________

Year_____________

Goal

Day														
1														
2														
3														
4														
5														
6														
7														

Daily Habit Tracker

Small Steps Lead To Big Results

Month ______________

Year ______________

Goal

Day
1
2
3
4
5
6
7

Daily Habit Tracker

Small Steps Lead To Big Results

Month_______________

Year_______________

Goal

Day															
1															
2															
3															
4															
5															
6															
7															

Daily Habit Tracker

Small Steps Lead To Big Results

Month ______________

Year ______________

Goal

Day															
1															
2															
3															
4															
5															
6															
7															

Daily Habit Tracker

Small Steps Lead To Big Results

Month ______________

Year ______________

Goal

Day															
1															
2															
3															
4															
5															
6															
7															

Daily Habit Tracker

Small Steps Lead To Big Results

Month

Year

Goal

Day														
1														
2														
3														
4														
5														
6														
7														

Daily Habit Tracker
Small Steps Lead To Big Results

Month______________

Year______________

Goal

Day															
1															
2															
3															
4															
5															
6															
7															

Daily Habit Tracker

Small Steps Lead To Big Results

Month ___________

Year ___________

Goal

Day														
1														
2														
3														
4														
5														
6														
7														

Daily Habit Tracker
Small Steps Lead To Big Results

Month _______________

Year _______________

Goal

Day															
1															
2															
3															
4															
5															
6															
7															

Daily Habit Tracker

Small Steps Lead To Big Results

Month________________

Year________________

Goal

Day														
1														
2														
3														
4														
5														
6														
7														

Daily Habit Tracker

Small Steps Lead To Big Results

Month_______________

Year_______________

Goal

Day														
1														
2														
3														
4														
5														
6														
7														

Daily Habit Tracker

Small Steps Lead To Big Results

Month______________

Year______________

Goal

Day														
1														
2														
3														
4														
5														
6														
7														

Daily Habit Tracker

Small Steps Lead To Big Results

Month

Year

Goal

Day														
1														
2														
3														
4														
5														
6														
7														

Daily Habit Tracker

Small Steps Lead To Big Results

Month______________

Year______________

Goal

Day														
1														
2														
3														
4														
5														
6														
7														

Daily Habit Tracker

Small Steps Lead To Big Results

Month_______________

Year_______________

Goal

Day															
1															
2															
3															
4															
5															
6															
7															

Daily Habit Tracker

Small Steps Lead To Big Results

Month

Year

Goal

Day																
1																
2																
3																
4																
5																
6																
7																

Daily Habit Tracker

Small Steps Lead To Big Results

Month________________

Year________________

Goal

Day															
1															
2															
3															
4															
5															
6															
7															

Daily Habit Tracker

Small Steps Lead To Big Results

Month_____________

Year_____________

Goal

Day															
1															
2															
3															
4															
5															
6															
7															

Daily Habit Tracker
Small Steps Lead To Big Results

Month______________

Year______________

Goal

Day														
1														
2														
3														
4														
5														
6														
7														

Daily Habit Tracker

Small Steps Lead To Big Results

Month_____________

Year_____________

Goal

Day														
1														
2														
3														
4														
5														
6														
7														

Daily Habit Tracker

Small Steps Lead To Big Results

Month _______________

Year _______________

Goal

Day														
1														
2														
3														
4														
5														
6														
7														

Daily Habit Tracker

Small Steps Lead To Big Results

Month_____________

Year_____________

Goal

Day														
1														
2														
3														
4														
5														
6														
7														

Daily Habit Tracker

Small Steps Lead To Big Results

Month ______________

Year ______________

Goal

Day													
1													
2													
3													
4													
5													
6													
7													

Daily Habit Tracker

Small Steps Lead To Big Results

Month ___________

Year ___________

Goal

Day															
1															
2															
3															
4															
5															
6															
7															

Daily Habit Tracker

Small Steps Lead To Big Results

Month _______________

Year _______________

Goal

Day															
1															
2															
3															
4															
5															
6															
7															

Daily Habit Tracker

Small Steps Lead To Big Results

Month _______________

Year _______________

Goal

Day															
1															
2															
3															
4															
5															
6															
7															

Daily Habit Tracker

Small Steps Lead To Big Results

Month ___________

Year ___________

Goal

Day															
1															
2															
3															
4															
5															
6															
7															

Daily Habit Tracker

Small Steps Lead To Big Results

Month_______________

Year_______________

Goal

Day														
1														
2														
3														
4														
5														
6														
7														

Daily Habit Tracker

Small Steps Lead To Big Results

Month _______________

Year _______________

Goal

Day														
1														
2														
3														
4														
5														
6														
7														

Daily Habit Tracker

Small Steps Lead To Big Results

Month _______________

Year _______________

Goal

Day															
1															
2															
3															
4															
5															
6															
7															

Daily Habit Tracker

Small Steps Lead To Big Results

Month_____________

Year_____________

Goal

Day														
1														
2														
3														
4														
5														
6														
7														

Daily Habit Tracker

Small Steps Lead To Big Results

Month___________

Year___________

Goal

Day													
1													
2													
3													
4													
5													
6													
7													

Daily Habit Tracker

Small Steps Lead To Big Results

Month ___________

Year ___________

Goal

Day															
1															
2															
3															
4															
5															
6															
7															

Daily Habit Tracker

Small Steps Lead To Big Results

Month_______________

Year_______________

Goal

Day															
1															
2															
3															
4															
5															
6															
7															

Daily Habit Tracker

Small Steps Lead To Big Results

Month ______________

Year ______________

Goal

Day														
1														
2														
3														
4														
5														
6														
7														

Daily Habit Tracker

Small Steps Lead To Big Results

Month ________________

Year ________________

Goal

Day														
1														
2														
3														
4														
5														
6														
7														

Daily Habit Tracker

Small Steps Lead To Big Results

Month______________

Year______________

Goal

Day														
1														
2														
3														
4														
5														
6														
7														

Daily Habit Tracker

Small Steps Lead To Big Results

Month _____________

Year _____________

Goal

Day															
1															
2															
3															
4															
5															
6															
7															

Daily Habit Tracker

Small Steps Lead To Big Results

Month ___________

Year ___________

Goal

Day														
1														
2														
3														
4														
5														
6														
7														

Daily Habit Tracker

Small Steps Lead To Big Results

Month_______________

Year_______________

Goal

Day

1

2

3

4

5

6

7

Daily Habit Tracker

Small Steps Lead To Big Results

Month _______________

Year _______________

Goal

Day														
1														
2														
3														
4														
5														
6														
7														

Daily Habit Tracker

Small Steps Lead To Big Results

Month ___________

Year ___________

Goal

Day

1

2

3

4

5

6

7

Daily Habit Tracker

Small Steps Lead To Big Results

Month _______________

Year _______________

Goal

Day															
1															
2															
3															
4															
5															
6															
7															

Daily Habit Tracker

Small Steps Lead To Big Results

Month _______________

Year _______________

Goal

Day															
1															
2															
3															
4															
5															
6															
7															

Daily Habit Tracker

Small Steps Lead To Big Results

Month _______________

Year _______________

Goal

Day															
1															
2															
3															
4															
5															
6															
7															

Daily Habit Tracker

Small Steps Lead To Big Results

Month______________

Year______________

Goal

Day														
1														
2														
3														
4														
5														
6														
7														

Daily Habit Tracker

Small Steps Lead To Big Results

Month _______________

Year _______________

Goal

Day														
1														
2														
3														
4														
5														
6														
7														

Daily Habit Tracker

Small Steps Lead To Big Results

Month _______________

Year _______________

Goal

Day														
1														
2														
3														
4														
5														
6														
7														

Daily Habit Tracker

Small Steps Lead To Big Results

Month_______________

Year_______________

Goal

Day														
1														
2														
3														
4														
5														
6														
7														

Daily Habit Tracker

Small Steps Lead To Big Results

Month _______________

Year _______________

Goal

Day															
1															
2															
3															
4															
5															
6															
7															

Daily Habit Tracker

Small Steps Lead To Big Results

Month_____________

Year_____________

Goal

Day														
1														
2														
3														
4														
5														
6														
7														

Daily Habit Tracker

Small Steps Lead To Big Results

Month_____________

Year_____________

Goal

Day														
1														
2														
3														
4														
5														
6														
7														

Daily Habit Tracker

Small Steps Lead To Big Results

Month ___________

Year ___________

Goal

Day														
1														
2														
3														
4														
5														
6														
7														

Daily Habit Tracker

Small Steps Lead To Big Results

Goal

Month_______________

Year_______________

Day	Goal													
1														
2														
3														
4														
5														
6														
7														

Daily Habit Tracker

Small Steps Lead To Big Results

Month______________

Year______________

Goal

Day																
1																
2																
3																
4																
5																
6																
7																

Daily Habit Tracker

Small Steps Lead To Big Results

Month __________

Year __________

Goal

Day														
1														
2														
3														
4														
5														
6														
7														

Daily Habit Tracker

Small Steps Lead To Big Results

Month

Year

Goal

Day															
1															
2															
3															
4															
5															
6															
7															

Daily Habit Tracker

Small Steps Lead To Big Results

Month_____________

Year_____________

Goal

Day															
1															
2															
3															
4															
5															
6															
7															

Daily Habit Tracker

Small Steps Lead To Big Results

Month ___________

Year ___________

Goal

Day															
1															
2															
3															
4															
5															
6															
7															

Daily Habit Tracker

Small Steps Lead To Big Results

Month

Year

Goal

Day

1

2

3

4

5

6

7

Daily Habit Tracker
Small Steps Lead To Big Results

Month______________

Year______________

Goal

Day															
1															
2															
3															
4															
5															
6															
7															

Daily Habit Tracker
Small Steps Lead To Big Results

Month ___________

Year ___________

Goal

Day														
1														
2														
3														
4														
5														
6														
7														

Daily Habit Tracker

Small Steps Lead To Big Results

Month _______________

Year _______________

Goal													
Day 1													
2													
3													
4													
5													
6													
7													

Daily Habit Tracker

Small Steps Lead To Big Results

Month_______________

Year_______________

Goal

Day														
1														
2														
3														
4														
5														
6														
7														

Daily Habit Tracker

Small Steps Lead To Big Results

Month________________

Year________________

Goal

Day															
1															
2															
3															
4															
5															
6															
7															

Daily Habit Tracker
Small Steps Lead To Big Results

Month______________

Year______________

Goal

Day													
1													
2													
3													
4													
5													
6													
7													

Daily Habit Tracker

Small Steps Lead To Big Results

Month________________

Year________________

Goal

Day														
1														
2														
3														
4														
5														
6														
7														

Daily Habit Tracker

Small Steps Lead To Big Results

Month_______________

Year_______________

Goal

Day
1
2
3
4
5
6
7

Daily Habit Tracker

Small Steps Lead To Big Results

Month_______________

Year_______________

Goal

Day															
1															
2															
3															
4															
5															
6															
7															

Daily Habit Tracker
Small Steps Lead To Big Results

Month ___________

Year ___________

Goal

Day														
1														
2														
3														
4														
5														
6														
7														

Daily Habit Tracker

Small Steps Lead To Big Results

Month ___________

Year ___________

Goal

Day														
1														
2														
3														
4														
5														
6														
7														

Daily Habit Tracker

Small Steps Lead To Big Results

Month______________

Year______________

Goal

Day														
1														
2														
3														
4														
5														
6														
7														

Daily Habit Tracker

Small Steps Lead To Big Results

Month _______________

Year _______________

Goal

Day														
1														
2														
3														
4														
5														
6														
7														

Daily Habit Tracker

Small Steps Lead To Big Results

Month_____________

Year_____________

Goal

Day															
1															
2															
3															
4															
5															
6															
7															

Daily Habit Tracker

Small Steps Lead To Big Results

Month_____________

Year_____________

Goal

Day														
1														
2														
3														
4														
5														
6														
7														

Daily Habit Tracker

Small Steps Lead To Big Results

Goal

Month _______________

Year _______________

Day															
1															
2															
3															
4															
5															
6															
7															

Daily Habit Tracker

Small Steps Lead To Big Results

Month ______________

Year ______________

Goal

Day														
1														
2														
3														
4														
5														
6														
7														

Daily Habit Tracker

Small Steps Lead To Big Results

Month _______________

Year _______________

Goal

Day															
1															
2															
3															
4															
5															
6															
7															

Daily Habit Tracker

Small Steps Lead To Big Results

Month _______________

Year _______________

Goal

Day															
1															
2															
3															
4															
5															
6															
7															

Daily Habit Tracker

Small Steps Lead To Big Results

Month _______________

Year _______________

Goal

Day														
1														
2														
3														
4														
5														
6														
7														

Daily Habit Tracker

Small Steps Lead To Big Results

Month_______________

Year_______________

Goal

Day														
1														
2														
3														
4														
5														
6														
7														

Daily Habit Tracker
Small Steps Lead To Big Results

Month ______________

Year ______________

Goal

Day														
1														
2														
3														
4														
5														
6														
7														

Daily Habit Tracker

Small Steps Lead To Big Results

Month __________

Year __________

Goal

Day															
1															
2															
3															
4															
5															
6															
7															

Daily Habit Tracker

Small Steps Lead To Big Results

Month _______________

Year _______________

Goal

Day															
1															
2															
3															
4															
5															
6															
7															

Daily Habit Tracker

Small Steps Lead To Big Results

Month ___________

Year ___________

Goal

Day															
1															
2															
3															
4															
5															
6															
7															

Daily Habit Tracker
Small Steps Lead To Big Results

Month ______________

Year ______________

Goal

Day														
1														
2														
3														
4														
5														
6														
7														

Daily Habit Tracker

Small Steps Lead To Big Results

Month __________

Year __________

Goal

Day															
1															
2															
3															
4															
5															
6															
7															

Daily Habit Tracker

Small Steps Lead To Big Results

Goal

Month ______________

Year ______________

Day														
1														
2														
3														
4														
5														
6														
7														

Daily Habit Tracker

Small Steps Lead To Big Results

Month _______________

Year _______________

Goal

Day															
1															
2															
3															
4															
5															
6															
7															

Daily Habit Tracker

Small Steps Lead To Big Results

Month_______________

Year_______________

Goal

Day															
1															
2															
3															
4															
5															
6															
7															

Daily Habit Tracker

Small Steps Lead To Big Results

Month____________

Year____________

Goal

Day														
1														
2														
3														
4														
5														
6														
7														

Daily Habit Tracker
Small Steps Lead To Big Results

Month _______________

Year _______________

Goal

Day															
1															
2															
3															
4															
5															
6															
7															

Daily Habit Tracker

Small Steps Lead To Big Results

Month ______________

Year ______________

Goal

Day														
1														
2														
3														
4														
5														
6														
7														

Daily Habit Tracker

Small Steps Lead To Big Results

Month

Year

Goal

Day														
1														
2														
3														
4														
5														
6														
7														

Daily Habit Tracker

Small Steps Lead To Big Results

Goal

Month ___________

Year ___________

Day															
1															
2															
3															
4															
5															
6															
7															

Daily Habit Tracker

Small Steps Lead To Big Results

Month _______________

Year _______________

Goal

Day															
1															
2															
3															
4															
5															
6															
7															

Daily Habit Tracker

Small Steps Lead To Big Results

Month __________

Year __________

Goal

Day															
1															
2															
3															
4															
5															
6															
7															

Daily Habit Tracker
Small Steps Lead To Big Results

Month________________

Year________________

Goal

Day															
1															
2															
3															
4															
5															
6															
7															

Daily Habit Tracker
Small Steps Lead To Big Results

Month _______________

Year _______________

Goal

Day													
1													
2													
3													
4													
5													
6													
7													

Daily Habit Tracker

Small Steps Lead To Big Results

Month_____________

Year_____________

Goal

Day															
1															
2															
3															
4															
5															
6															
7															

Daily Habit Tracker

Small Steps Lead To Big Results

Month ___________

Year ___________

Goal

Day															
1															
2															
3															
4															
5															
6															
7															

Daily Habit Tracker

Small Steps Lead To Big Results

Month _____________

Year _____________

Goal

Day															
1															
2															
3															
4															
5															
6															
7															

Daily Habit Tracker

Small Steps Lead To Big Results

Month _______________

Year _______________

Goal

Day														
1														
2														
3														
4														
5														
6														
7														

Daily Habit Tracker

Small Steps Lead To Big Results

Month ______________

Year ______________

Goal

Day															
1															
2															
3															
4															
5															
6															
7															

Daily Habit Tracker
Small Steps Lead To Big Results

Month _______________

Year _______________

Goal

Day															
1															
2															
3															
4															
5															
6															
7															

Daily Habit Tracker

Small Steps Lead To Big Results

Month ___________

Year ___________

Goal

Day															
1															
2															
3															
4															
5															
6															
7															

Daily Habit Tracker

Small Steps Lead To Big Results

Month ___________

Year ___________

Goal

Day															
1															
2															
3															
4															
5															
6															
7															

Daily Habit Tracker

Small Steps Lead To Big Results

Month _______________

Year _______________

Goal

Day														
1														
2														
3														
4														
5														
6														
7														

Daily Habit Tracker

Small Steps Lead To Big Results

Month __________

Year __________

Goal

Day															
1															
2															
3															
4															
5															
6															
7															

Daily Habit Tracker

Small Steps Lead To Big Results

Month

Year

Goal

Day															
1															
2															
3															
4															
5															
6															
7															

Daily Habit Tracker

Small Steps Lead To Big Results

Month

Year

Goal

Day															
1															
2															
3															
4															
5															
6															
7															

Daily Habit Tracker

Small Steps Lead To Big Results

Month ___________

Year ___________

Goal

Day														
1														
2														
3														
4														
5														
6														
7														

Daily Habit Tracker

Small Steps Lead To Big Results

Month _______________

Year _______________

Goal

Day															
1															
2															
3															
4															
5															
6															
7															

Daily Habit Tracker

Small Steps Lead To Big Results

Month_____________

Year_____________

Goal

Day															
1															
2															
3															
4															
5															
6															
7															

Daily Habit Tracker

Small Steps Lead To Big Results

Month

Year

Goal

Day													
1													
2													
3													
4													
5													
6													
7													

Daily Habit Tracker
Small Steps Lead To Big Results

Month________________

Year________________

Goal

Day														
1														
2														
3														
4														
5														
6														
7														

Daily Habit Tracker

Small Steps Lead To Big Results

Month______________

Year______________

Goal

Day															
1															
2															
3															
4															
5															
6															
7															

Daily Habit Tracker

Small Steps Lead To Big Results

Month ___________

Year ___________

Goal

Day															
1															
2															
3															
4															
5															
6															
7															

Daily Habit Tracker

Small Steps Lead To Big Results

Month ___________

Year ___________

Goal

Day													
1													
2													
3													
4													
5													
6													
7													

Daily Habit Tracker

Small Steps Lead To Big Results

Month ___________

Year ___________

Goal

Day														
1														
2														
3														
4														
5														
6														
7														

Daily Habit Tracker

Small Steps Lead To Big Results

Month ______________

Year ______________

Goal

Day															
1															
2															
3															
4															
5															
6															
7															

Daily Habit Tracker

Small Steps Lead To Big Results

Month _______________

Year _______________

Goal

Day														
1														
2														
3														
4														
5														
6														
7														

Daily Habit Tracker

Small Steps Lead To Big Results

Month__________

Year__________

Goal

Day														
1														
2														
3														
4														
5														
6														
7														

Daily Habit Tracker

Small Steps Lead To Big Results

Month ___________

Year ___________

Goal

Day														
1														
2														
3														
4														
5														
6														
7														

Daily Habit Tracker

Small Steps Lead To Big Results

Month ___________

Year ___________

Goal

Day															
1															
2															
3															
4															
5															
6															
7															

Daily Habit Tracker

Small Steps Lead To Big Results

Month_______________

Year_______________

Goal

Day															
1															
2															
3															
4															
5															
6															
7															

Daily Habit Tracker

Small Steps Lead To Big Results

Month __________

Year __________

Goal

Day														
1														
2														
3														
4														
5														
6														
7														

Daily Habit Tracker

Small Steps Lead To Big Results

Month_____________

Year_____________

Goal

Day															
1															
2															
3															
4															
5															
6															
7															

Daily Habit Tracker

Small Steps Lead To Big Results

Month________________

Year________________

Goal

Day														
1														
2														
3														
4														
5														
6														
7														

Daily Habit Tracker

Small Steps Lead To Big Results

Month_______________

Year_______________

Goal

Day														
1														
2														
3														
4														
5														
6														
7														

Daily Habit Tracker

Small Steps Lead To Big Results

Month ___________

Year ___________

Goal

Day														
1														
2														
3														
4														
5														
6														
7														

Daily Habit Tracker

Small Steps Lead To Big Results

Month _______________

Year _______________

Goal

Day														
1														
2														
3														
4														
5														
6														
7														

Daily Habit Tracker

Small Steps Lead To Big Results

Month_______________

Year_______________

Goal

Day															
1															
2															
3															
4															
5															
6															
7															

Daily Habit Tracker

Small Steps Lead To Big Results

Month______________

Year______________

Goal

Day															
1															
2															
3															
4															
5															
6															
7															

Daily Habit Tracker

Small Steps Lead To Big Results

Month_____________

Year_____________

Goal

Day															
1															
2															
3															
4															
5															
6															
7															

Daily Habit Tracker

Small Steps Lead To Big Results

Month ____________

Year ____________

Goal

Day															
1															
2															
3															
4															
5															
6															
7															

Daily Habit Tracker

Small Steps Lead To Big Results

Month

Year

Goal

Day															
1															
2															
3															
4															
5															
6															
7															

Daily Habit Tracker

Small Steps Lead To Big Results

Month _______________

Year _______________

Goal

Day														
1														
2														
3														
4														
5														
6														
7														

Daily Habit Tracker

Small Steps Lead To Big Results

Month ___________

Year ___________

Goal

Day														
1														
2														
3														
4														
5														
6														
7														

Daily Habit Tracker

Small Steps Lead To Big Results

Month __________

Year __________

Goal

Day															
1															
2															
3															
4															
5															
6															
7															

Daily Habit Tracker

Small Steps Lead To Big Results

Month_____________

Year_____________

Goal

Day													
1													
2													
3													
4													
5													
6													
7													

Daily Habit Tracker

Small Steps Lead To Big Results

Month ______________

Year ______________

Goal

Day														
1														
2														
3														
4														
5														
6														
7														

Daily Habit Tracker

Small Steps Lead To Big Results

Month _______________

Year _______________

Goal

Day														
1														
2														
3														
4														
5														
6														
7														

Daily Habit Tracker

Small Steps Lead To Big Results

Month _______________

Year _______________

Goal														
Day 1														
2														
3														
4														
5														
6														
7														

Daily Habit Tracker

Small Steps Lead To Big Results

Month______________

Year______________

Goal

Day														
1														
2														
3														
4														
5														
6														
7														

Daily Habit Tracker

Small Steps Lead To Big Results

Month_______________

Year_______________

Goal

Day														
1														
2														
3														
4														
5														
6														
7														

Daily Habit Tracker

Small Steps Lead To Big Results

Month _______________

Year _______________

Goal

Day														
1														
2														
3														
4														
5														
6														
7														

Daily Habit Tracker

Small Steps Lead To Big Results

Month

Year

Goal

Day

1

2

3

4

5

6

7

Daily Habit Tracker
Small Steps Lead To Big Results

Month __________

Year __________

Goal

Day																
1																
2																
3																
4																
5																
6																
7																

Daily Habit Tracker

Small Steps Lead To Big Results

Month ______________

Year ______________

Goal

Day														
1														
2														
3														
4														
5														
6														
7														

Daily Habit Tracker

Small Steps Lead To Big Results

Month ________________

Year ________________

Goal

Day															
1															
2															
3															
4															
5															
6															
7															

Daily Habit Tracker

Small Steps Lead To Big Results

Month_______________

Year_______________

Goal

Day														
1														
2														
3														
4														
5														
6														
7														

Daily Habit Tracker

Small Steps Lead To Big Results

Month _______________

Year _______________

Goal

Day															
1															
2															
3															
4															
5															
6															
7															

Daily Habit Tracker

Small Steps Lead To Big Results

Month ___________

Year ___________

Goal

Day														
1														
2														
3														
4														
5														
6														
7														

Daily Habit Tracker

Small Steps Lead To Big Results

Month_______________

Year_______________

Goal

Day															
1															
2															
3															
4															
5															
6															
7															

Daily Habit Tracker

Small Steps Lead To Big Results

Month ___________

Year ___________

Goal

Day															
1															
2															
3															
4															
5															
6															
7															

Daily Habit Tracker

Small Steps Lead To Big Results

Month __________

Year __________

Goal

Day

1

2

3

4

5

6

7

Daily Habit Tracker

Small Steps Lead To Big Results

Month __________

Year __________

Goal

Day															
1															
2															
3															
4															
5															
6															
7															

Daily Habit Tracker

Small Steps Lead To Big Results

Month _______________

Year _______________

Goal

Day														
1														
2														
3														
4														
5														
6														
7														

Daily Habit Tracker

Small Steps Lead To Big Results

Month ________________

Year ________________

Goal

Day														
1														
2														
3														
4														
5														
6														
7														

Daily Habit Tracker

Small Steps Lead To Big Results

Month_____________

Year_____________

Goal

Day														
1														
2														
3														
4														
5														
6														
7														

Daily Habit Tracker

Small Steps Lead To Big Results

Month __________

Year __________

Goal

Day														
1														
2														
3														
4														
5														
6														
7														

Daily Habit Tracker

Small Steps Lead To Big Results

Month_______________

Year_______________

Goal

Day															
1															
2															
3															
4															
5															
6															
7															

Daily Habit Tracker

Small Steps Lead To Big Results

Month_____________

Year_____________

Goal

Day															
1															
2															
3															
4															
5															
6															
7															

Daily Habit Tracker

Small Steps Lead To Big Results

Month _______________

Year _______________

Goal

Day															
1															
2															
3															
4															
5															
6															
7															

Daily Habit Tracker

Small Steps Lead To Big Results

Month

Year

Goal

Day														
1														
2														
3														
4														
5														
6														
7														

Daily Habit Tracker

Small Steps Lead To Big Results

Month __________

Year __________

Goal

Day														
1														
2														
3														
4														
5														
6														
7														

Daily Habit Tracker

Small Steps Lead To Big Results

Month _______________

Year _______________

Goal

Day														
1														
2														
3														
4														
5														
6														
7														

Daily Habit Tracker

Small Steps Lead To Big Results

Month _______________

Year _______________

Goal

Day															
1															
2															
3															
4															
5															
6															
7															

Daily Habit Tracker

Small Steps Lead To Big Results

Month________________

Year________________

Goal

Day															
1															
2															
3															
4															
5															
6															
7															

Daily Habit Tracker

Small Steps Lead To Big Results

Month ___________

Year ___________

Goal

Day														
1														
2														
3														
4														
5														
6														
7														

Daily Habit Tracker
Small Steps Lead To Big Results

Month __________

Year __________

Goal

Day															
1															
2															
3															
4															
5															
6															
7															

Daily Habit Tracker

Small Steps Lead To Big Results

Month ________________

Year ________________

Goal

Day														
1														
2														
3														
4														
5														
6														
7														

Daily Habit Tracker

Small Steps Lead To Big Results

Month

Year

Goal

Day														
1														
2														
3														
4														
5														
6														
7														

Daily Habit Tracker

Small Steps Lead To Big Results

Month ___________

Year ___________

Goal

Day

1

2

3

4

5

6

7

Daily Habit Tracker

Small Steps Lead To Big Results

Month ___________

Year ___________

Goal

Day														
1														
2														
3														
4														
5														
6														
7														

Daily Habit Tracker

Small Steps Lead To Big Results

Month ______

Year ______

Goal

Day														
1														
2														
3														
4														
5														
6														
7														

Daily Habit Tracker
Small Steps Lead To Big Results

Month______________

Year______________

Goal

Day															
1															
2															
3															
4															
5															
6															
7															

Daily Habit Tracker

Small Steps Lead To Big Results

Month______________

Year______________

Goal

Day													
1													
2													
3													
4													
5													
6													
7													

Daily Habit Tracker

Small Steps Lead To Big Results

Month ______________

Year ______________

Goal

Day															
1															
2															
3															
4															
5															
6															
7															

Daily Habit Tracker

Small Steps Lead To Big Results

Month _______________

Year _______________

Goal

Day														
1														
2														
3														
4														
5														
6														
7														

Daily Habit Tracker

Small Steps Lead To Big Results

Month_____________

Year_____________

Goal

Day														
1														
2														
3														
4														
5														
6														
7														

Daily Habit Tracker

Small Steps Lead To Big Results

Month ______________________

Year ______________________

Goal

Day														
1														
2														
3														
4														
5														
6														
7														

Daily Habit Tracker

Small Steps Lead To Big Results

Month _______________

Year _______________

Goal

Day															
1															
2															
3															
4															
5															
6															
7															

Daily Habit Tracker

Small Steps Lead To Big Results

Month_______________

Year_______________

Goal

Day																
1																
2																
3																
4																
5																
6																
7																

Daily Habit Tracker

Small Steps Lead To Big Results

Month _____________

Year _____________

Goal

Day															
1															
2															
3															
4															
5															
6															
7															

Daily Habit Tracker

Small Steps Lead To Big Results

Month______________

Year______________

Goal

Day																
1																
2																
3																
4																
5																
6																
7																

Daily Habit Tracker

Small Steps Lead To Big Results

Month________________

Year________________

Goal

Day															
1															
2															
3															
4															
5															
6															
7															

Daily Habit Tracker

Small Steps Lead To Big Results

Month _____________

Year _____________

Goal

Day															
1															
2															
3															
4															
5															
6															
7															

Daily Habit Tracker

Small Steps Lead To Big Results

Month _______________

Year _______________

Goal

Day														
1														
2														
3														
4														
5														
6														
7														

Daily Habit Tracker

Small Steps Lead To Big Results

Month_____________

Year_____________

Goal

Day															
1															
2															
3															
4															
5															
6															
7															

Daily Habit Tracker

Small Steps Lead To Big Results

Month _______________

Year _______________

Goal

Day														
1														
2														
3														
4														
5														
6														
7														

Daily Habit Tracker

Small Steps Lead To Big Results

Month ___________

Year ___________

Goal

Day															
1															
2															
3															
4															
5															
6															
7															

Daily Habit Tracker

Small Steps Lead To Big Results

Month _______________

Year _______________

Goal

Day														
1														
2														
3														
4														
5														
6														
7														

Daily Habit Tracker

Small Steps Lead To Big Results

Month ______________

Year ______________

Goal

Day															
1															
2															
3															
4															
5															
6															
7															

Daily Habit Tracker

Small Steps Lead To Big Results

Month

Year

Goal

Day															
1															
2															
3															
4															
5															
6															
7															

Daily Habit Tracker

Small Steps Lead To Big Results

Month________

Year________

Goal

Day															
1															
2															
3															
4															
5															
6															
7															

Daily Habit Tracker

Small Steps Lead To Big Results

Month ___________

Year ___________

Goal

Day														
1														
2														
3														
4														
5														
6														
7														

Daily Habit Tracker

Small Steps Lead To Big Results

Month _______________

Year _______________

Goal

Day														
1														
2														
3														
4														
5														
6														
7														

Daily Habit Tracker

Small Steps Lead To Big Results

Month________________

Year________________

Goal

Day														
1														
2														
3														
4														
5														
6														
7														

Daily Habit Tracker

Small Steps Lead To Big Results

Month __________

Year __________

Goal

Day														
1														
2														
3														
4														
5														
6														
7														

Daily Habit Tracker

Small Steps Lead To Big Results

Month _______________

Year _______________

Goal

Day													
1													
2													
3													
4													
5													
6													
7													

Daily Habit Tracker

Small Steps Lead To Big Results

Month_______________

Year_______________

Goal

Day														
1														
2														
3														
4														
5														
6														
7														

Daily Habit Tracker

Small Steps Lead To Big Results

Month _______________

Year _______________

Goal

Day														
1														
2														
3														
4														
5														
6														
7														

Daily Habit Tracker

Small Steps Lead To Big Results

Month_______________

Year_______________

Goal

Day															
1															
2															
3															
4															
5															
6															
7															

Daily Habit Tracker

Small Steps Lead To Big Results

Month ___________

Year ___________

Goal

Day															
1															
2															
3															
4															
5															
6															
7															

Daily Habit Tracker

Small Steps Lead To Big Results

Month

Year

Goal

Day														
1														
2														
3														
4														
5														
6														
7														

Daily Habit Tracker
Small Steps Lead To Big Results

Month_______________

Year_______________

Goal

Day													
1													
2													
3													
4													
5													
6													
7													

Daily Habit Tracker

Small Steps Lead To Big Results

Month_______________

Year_______________

Goal

Day														
1														
2														
3														
4														
5														
6														
7														

Daily Habit Tracker

Small Steps Lead To Big Results

Month ___________

Year ___________

Goal

Day															
1															
2															
3															
4															
5															
6															
7															

Daily Habit Tracker

Small Steps Lead To Big Results

Month ________________

Year ________________

Goal

Day															
1															
2															
3															
4															
5															
6															
7															

Daily Habit Tracker

Small Steps Lead To Big Results

Month_______________

Year_______________

Goal

Day														
1														
2														
3														
4														
5														
6														
7														

Daily Habit Tracker

Small Steps Lead To Big Results

Goal

Month_____________

Year_____________

Day

1

2

3

4

5

6

7

Daily Habit Tracker

Small Steps Lead To Big Results

Month _______________

Year _______________

Goal

Day														
1														
2														
3														
4														
5														
6														
7														

Daily Habit Tracker

Small Steps Lead To Big Results

Month ______________

Year ______________

Goal

Day															
1															
2															
3															
4															
5															
6															
7															

Daily Habit Tracker

Small Steps Lead To Big Results

Month ______________

Year ______________

Goal

Day															
1															
2															
3															
4															
5															
6															
7															

Daily Habit Tracker

Small Steps Lead To Big Results

Month ___________

Year ___________

Goal

Day														
1														
2														
3														
4														
5														
6														
7														

Daily Habit Tracker

Small Steps Lead To Big Results

Month_______________

Year_______________

Goal

Day														
1														
2														
3														
4														
5														
6														
7														

Daily Habit Tracker

Small Steps Lead To Big Results

Month

Year

Goal

Day														
1														
2														
3														
4														
5														
6														
7														

Daily Habit Tracker

Small Steps Lead To Big Results

Month ___________

Year ___________

Goal

Day														
1														
2														
3														
4														
5														
6														
7														

Daily Habit Tracker

Small Steps Lead To Big Results

Goal

Month ___________

Year ___________

Day														
1														
2														
3														
4														
5														
6														
7														

Daily Habit Tracker

Small Steps Lead To Big Results

Month ____________________

Year ____________________

Goal

Day															
1															
2															
3															
4															
5															
6															
7															

Daily Habit Tracker

Small Steps Lead To Big Results

Month ______________

Year ______________

Goal

Day														
1														
2														
3														
4														
5														
6														
7														

Daily Habit Tracker
Small Steps Lead To Big Results

Month_____________

Year_____________

Goal

Day															
1															
2															
3															
4															
5															
6															
7															

Daily Habit Tracker

Small Steps Lead To Big Results

Month________________

Year________________

Goal

Day														
1														
2														
3														
4														
5														
6														
7														

Daily Habit Tracker
Small Steps Lead To Big Results

Month__________

Year__________

Goal

Day														
1														
2														
3														
4														
5														
6														
7														

Daily Habit Tracker

Small Steps Lead To Big Results

Month_______________

Year_______________

Goal

Day														
1														
2														
3														
4														
5														
6														
7														

Daily Habit Tracker

Small Steps Lead To Big Results

Month ___________

Year ___________

Goal

Day														
1														
2														
3														
4														
5														
6														
7														

Daily Habit Tracker

Small Steps Lead To Big Results

Month _______________

Year _______________

Goal

Day															
1															
2															
3															
4															
5															
6															
7															

Daily Habit Tracker
Small Steps Lead To Big Results

Month ___________

Year ___________

Goal

Day															
1															
2															
3															
4															
5															
6															
7															

Daily Habit Tracker

Small Steps Lead To Big Results

Month __________

Year __________

Goal

Day															
1															
2															
3															
4															
5															
6															
7															

Daily Habit Tracker

Small Steps Lead To Big Results

Month_______________

Year_______________

Goal

Day															
1															
2															
3															
4															
5															
6															
7															

Daily Habit Tracker
Small Steps Lead To Big Results

Month _______________

Year _______________

Goal

Day															
1															
2															
3															
4															
5															
6															
7															

Daily Habit Tracker

Small Steps Lead To Big Results

Month

Year

Goal

Day

1

2

3

4

5

6

7

Daily Habit Tracker

Small Steps Lead To Big Results

Month_______________

Year_______________

Goal

Day															
1															
2															
3															
4															
5															
6															
7															

Daily Habit Tracker

Small Steps Lead To Big Results

Month ___________

Year ___________

Goal

Day															
1															
2															
3															
4															
5															
6															
7															

Daily Habit Tracker

Small Steps Lead To Big Results

Month ______________________

Year ______________________

Goal

Day														
1														
2														
3														
4														
5														
6														
7														

Daily Habit Tracker

Small Steps Lead To Big Results

Month _______________

Year _______________

Goal

Day														
1														
2														
3														
4														
5														
6														
7														

Daily Habit Tracker

Small Steps Lead To Big Results

Month ______________

Year ______________

Goal

Day														
1														
2														
3														
4														
5														
6														
7														

Daily Habit Tracker

Small Steps Lead To Big Results

Month_____________

Year_____________

Goal

Day														
1														
2														
3														
4														
5														
6														
7														

Daily Habit Tracker

Small Steps Lead To Big Results

Month_______________

Year_______________

Goal

Day														
1														
2														
3														
4														
5														
6														
7														

Daily Habit Tracker
Small Steps Lead To Big Results

Month_______________

Year_______________

Goal

Day													
1													
2													
3													
4													
5													
6													
7													

Daily Habit Tracker

Small Steps Lead To Big Results

Month ___________

Year ___________

Goal

Day															
1															
2															
3															
4															
5															
6															
7															

Daily Habit Tracker

Small Steps Lead To Big Results

Month ___________

Year ___________

Goal

Day																
1																
2																
3																
4																
5																
6																
7																

Daily Habit Tracker

Small Steps Lead To Big Results

Month ______________

Year ______________

Goal

Day															
1															
2															
3															
4															
5															
6															
7															

Daily Habit Tracker

Small Steps Lead To Big Results

Month

Year

Goal

Day															
1															
2															
3															
4															
5															
6															
7															

Daily Habit Tracker

Small Steps Lead To Big Results

Month_______________

Year_______________

Goal

Day															
1															
2															
3															
4															
5															
6															
7															

Daily Habit Tracker

Small Steps Lead To Big Results

Month

Year

Goal

Day														
1														
2														
3														
4														
5														
6														
7														

Daily Habit Tracker

Small Steps Lead To Big Results

Month __________

Year __________

Goal

Day															
1															
2															
3															
4															
5															
6															
7															

Daily Habit Tracker

Small Steps Lead To Big Results

Month__________

Year__________

Goal

Day														
1														
2														
3														
4														
5														
6														
7														

Daily Habit Tracker

Small Steps Lead To Big Results

Month__________

Year__________

Goal

Day														
1														
2														
3														
4														
5														
6														
7														

Daily Habit Tracker

Small Steps Lead To Big Results

Month ___________________

Year ___________________

Goal

Day

1

2

3

4

5

6

7

Daily Habit Tracker

Small Steps Lead To Big Results

Month__________

Year__________

Goal

Day													
1													
2													
3													
4													
5													
6													
7													

Daily Habit Tracker

Small Steps Lead To Big Results

Month

Year

Goal

Day														
1														
2														
3														
4														
5														
6														
7														

Daily Habit Tracker

Small Steps Lead To Big Results

Month ______________

Year ______________

Goal

Day															
1															
2															
3															
4															
5															
6															
7															

Daily Habit Tracker

Small Steps Lead To Big Results

Month _______________

Year _______________

Goal

Day														
1														
2														
3														
4														
5														
6														
7														

Daily Habit Tracker

Small Steps Lead To Big Results

Month________________

Year________________

Goal

Day															
1															
2															
3															
4															
5															
6															
7															

Daily Habit Tracker

Small Steps Lead To Big Results

Month ________________

Year ________________

Goal

Day															
1															
2															
3															
4															
5															
6															
7															

Daily Habit Tracker

Small Steps Lead To Big Results

Month ___________

Year ___________

Goal

Day														
1														
2														
3														
4														
5														
6														
7														

Daily Habit Tracker

Small Steps Lead To Big Results

Month_____________

Year_____________

Goal

Day														
1														
2														
3														
4														
5														
6														
7														

Daily Habit Tracker

Small Steps Lead To Big Results

Month ______________________

Year ______________________

Goal

Day														
1														
2														
3														
4														
5														
6														
7														

Daily Habit Tracker
Small Steps Lead To Big Results

Month ___________

Year ___________

Goal

Day															
1															
2															
3															
4															
5															
6															
7															

Daily Habit Tracker

Small Steps Lead To Big Results

Goal

Month ______________

Year ______________

Day															
1															
2															
3															
4															
5															
6															
7															

Daily Habit Tracker

Small Steps Lead To Big Results

Month________________

Year________________

Goal

Day														
1														
2														
3														
4														
5														
6														
7														

Daily Habit Tracker

Small Steps Lead To Big Results

Month______________

Year______________

Goal

Day																
1																
2																
3																
4																
5																
6																
7																

Daily Habit Tracker

Small Steps Lead To Big Results

Month _______________

Year _______________

Goal

Day															
1															
2															
3															
4															
5															
6															
7															

Daily Habit Tracker

Small Steps Lead To Big Results

Month ___________

Year ___________

Goal

Day															
1															
2															
3															
4															
5															
6															
7															

Daily Habit Tracker

Small Steps Lead To Big Results

Month_____________

Year_____________

Goal

Day															
1															
2															
3															
4															
5															
6															
7															

Daily Habit Tracker

Small Steps Lead To Big Results

Month ____________

Year ____________

Goal

Day															
1															
2															
3															
4															
5															
6															
7															

Daily Habit Tracker

Small Steps Lead To Big Results

Month __________

Year __________

Goal

Day															
1															
2															
3															
4															
5															
6															
7															

Daily Habit Tracker

Small Steps Lead To Big Results

Month __________

Year __________

Goal

Day														
1														
2														
3														
4														
5														
6														
7														

Daily Habit Tracker

Small Steps Lead To Big Results

Month ________________

Year ________________

Goal

Day														
1														
2														
3														
4														
5														
6														
7														

Daily Habit Tracker

Small Steps Lead To Big Results

Month _______________

Year _______________

Goal

Day														
1														
2														
3														
4														
5														
6														
7														

Daily Habit Tracker

Small Steps Lead To Big Results

Month______________

Year______________

Goal

Day														
1														
2														
3														
4														
5														
6														
7														

Daily Habit Tracker

Small Steps Lead To Big Results

Month ___________

Year ___________

Goal

Day														
1														
2														
3														
4														
5														
6														
7														

Daily Habit Tracker

Small Steps Lead To Big Results

Month ___________

Year ___________

Goal

Day														
1														
2														
3														
4														
5														
6														
7														

Daily Habit Tracker

Small Steps Lead To Big Results

Month ______________

Year ______________

Goal

Day														
1														
2														
3														
4														
5														
6														
7														

Daily Habit Tracker

Small Steps Lead To Big Results

Month ________________

Year ________________

Goal

Day															
1															
2															
3															
4															
5															
6															
7															

Daily Habit Tracker

Small Steps Lead To Big Results

Month ___________

Year ___________

Goal

Day														
1														
2														
3														
4														
5														
6														
7														

Daily Habit Tracker

Small Steps Lead To Big Results

Month_______________

Year_______________

Goal

Day														
1														
2														
3														
4														
5														
6														
7														

Daily Habit Tracker

Small Steps Lead To Big Results

Month ______________

Year ______________

Goal

Day														
1														
2														
3														
4														
5														
6														
7														

Daily Habit Tracker
Small Steps Lead To Big Results

Month ___________

Year ___________

Goal

Day														
1														
2														
3														
4														
5														
6														
7														

Daily Habit Tracker

Small Steps Lead To Big Results

Month___________

Year___________

Goal

Day															
1															
2															
3															
4															
5															
6															
7															

Daily Habit Tracker

Small Steps Lead To Big Results

Month_______________

Year_______________

Goal

Day															
1															
2															
3															
4															
5															
6															
7															

Daily Habit Tracker

Small Steps Lead To Big Results

Month _______________

Year _______________

Goal

Day															
1															
2															
3															
4															
5															
6															
7															

Daily Habit Tracker

Small Steps Lead To Big Results

Month_______________

Year_______________

Goal

Day														
1														
2														
3														
4														
5														
6														
7														

Daily Habit Tracker

Small Steps Lead To Big Results

Month __________

Year __________

Goal

Day														
1														
2														
3														
4														
5														
6														
7														

Daily Habit Tracker

Small Steps Lead To Big Results

Month_____________

Year_____________

Goal

Day															
1															
2															
3															
4															
5															
6															
7															

Daily Habit Tracker

Small Steps Lead To Big Results

Month_______________

Year_______________

Goal

Day													
1													
2													
3													
4													
5													
6													
7													

Daily Habit Tracker

Small Steps Lead To Big Results

Month __________

Year __________

Goal

Day															
1															
2															
3															
4															
5															
6															
7															

Daily Habit Tracker

Small Steps Lead To Big Results

Month _______________

Year _______________

Goal

Day															
1															
2															
3															
4															
5															
6															
7															

Daily Habit Tracker

Small Steps Lead To Big Results

Month ___________

Year ___________

Goal

Day														
1														
2														
3														
4														
5														
6														
7														

Daily Habit Tracker

Small Steps Lead To Big Results

Month_______________

Year_______________

Goal

Day														
1														
2														
3														
4														
5														
6														
7														

Daily Habit Tracker

Small Steps Lead To Big Results

Month

Year

Goal

Day

1

2

3

4

5

6

7

Daily Habit Tracker

Small Steps Lead To Big Results

Month _______________

Year _______________

Goal

Day															
1															
2															
3															
4															
5															
6															
7															

Daily Habit Tracker

Small Steps Lead To Big Results

Month ___________

Year ___________

Goal

Day														
1														
2														
3														
4														
5														
6														
7														

Daily Habit Tracker

Small Steps Lead To Big Results

Month _______________

Year _______________

Goal

Day															
1															
2															
3															
4															
5															
6															
7															

Daily Habit Tracker

Small Steps Lead To Big Results

Month _______________

Year _______________

Goal

Day															
1															
2															
3															
4															
5															
6															
7															

Daily Habit Tracker

Small Steps Lead To Big Results

Month

Year

Goal

Day															
1															
2															
3															
4															
5															
6															
7															

Daily Habit Tracker

Small Steps Lead To Big Results

Month ________

Year ________

Goal

Day														
1														
2														
3														
4														
5														
6														
7														

Daily Habit Tracker

Small Steps Lead To Big Results

Month_______________

Year_______________

Goal

Day														
1														
2														
3														
4														
5														
6														
7														

Daily Habit Tracker

Small Steps Lead To Big Results

Month ___________

Year ___________

Goal

Day														
1														
2														
3														
4														
5														
6														
7														

Daily Habit Tracker
Small Steps Lead To Big Results

Month _______________

Year _______________

Goal

Day														
1														
2														
3														
4														
5														
6														
7														

Daily Habit Tracker

Small Steps Lead To Big Results

Month________________

Year________________

Goal

Day															
1															
2															
3															
4															
5															
6															
7															

Daily Habit Tracker

Small Steps Lead To Big Results

Month_____________

Year_____________

Goal

Day														
1														
2														
3														
4														
5														
6														
7														

Daily Habit Tracker

Small Steps Lead To Big Results

Month________________

Year________________

Goal

Day														
1														
2														
3														
4														
5														
6														
7														

Daily Habit Tracker

Small Steps Lead To Big Results

Month ______________

Year ______________

Goal

Day														
1														
2														
3														
4														
5														
6														
7														

Daily Habit Tracker

Small Steps Lead To Big Results

Month_______________

Year_______________

Goal

Day															
1															
2															
3															
4															
5															
6															
7															

Daily Habit Tracker

Small Steps Lead To Big Results

Month ______________

Year ______________

Goal

Day															
1															
2															
3															
4															
5															
6															
7															

Daily Habit Tracker

Small Steps Lead To Big Results

Month _______________

Year _______________

Goal

Day														
1														
2														
3														
4														
5														
6														
7														

Daily Habit Tracker

Small Steps Lead To Big Results

Month

Year

Goal

Day															
1															
2															
3															
4															
5															
6															
7															

Daily Habit Tracker

Small Steps Lead To Big Results

Month______________

Year______________

Goal

Day															
1															
2															
3															
4															
5															
6															
7															

Daily Habit Tracker

Small Steps Lead To Big Results

Month ___________

Year ___________

Goal

Day														
1														
2														
3														
4														
5														
6														
7														

Daily Habit Tracker

Small Steps Lead To Big Results

Month________________

Year________________

Goal

Day														
1														
2														
3														
4														
5														
6														
7														

Daily Habit Tracker

Small Steps Lead To Big Results

Month _______________

Year _______________

Goal

Day														
1														
2														
3														
4														
5														
6														
7														

Daily Habit Tracker
Small Steps Lead To Big Results

Month ___________

Year ___________

Day															
1															
2															
3															
4															
5															
6															
7															

Daily Habit Tracker

Small Steps Lead To Big Results

Month ______________

Year ______________

Goal

Day														
1														
2														
3														
4														
5														
6														
7														

Daily Habit Tracker

Small Steps Lead To Big Results

Month ______________

Year ______________

Goal

Day															
1															
2															
3															
4															
5															
6															
7															

Daily Habit Tracker

Small Steps Lead To Big Results

Month

Year

Goal

Day														
1														
2														
3														
4														
5														
6														
7														

Daily Habit Tracker
Small Steps Lead To Big Results

Month _______________

Year _______________

Goal

Day														
1														
2														
3														
4														
5														
6														
7														

Daily Habit Tracker

Small Steps Lead To Big Results

Month_____________

Year_____________

Goal

Day														
1														
2														
3														
4														
5														
6														
7														

Daily Habit Tracker
Small Steps Lead To Big Results

Month _______________

Year _______________

Goal

Day															
1															
2															
3															
4															
5															
6															
7															

Daily Habit Tracker

Small Steps Lead To Big Results

Month ______________

Year ______________

Goal

Day															
1															
2															
3															
4															
5															
6															
7															

Daily Habit Tracker

Small Steps Lead To Big Results

Month _______________

Year _______________

Goal

Day															
1															
2															
3															
4															
5															
6															
7															

Daily Habit Tracker

Small Steps Lead To Big Results

Month ____________

Year ____________

Goal

Day															
1															
2															
3															
4															
5															
6															
7															

Daily Habit Tracker

Small Steps Lead To Big Results

Month ___________

Year ___________

Goal

Day														
1														
2														
3														
4														
5														
6														
7														

Daily Habit Tracker

Small Steps Lead To Big Results

Month _______________

Year _______________

Goal

Day														
1														
2														
3														
4														
5														
6														
7														

Daily Habit Tracker

Small Steps Lead To Big Results

Month __________

Year __________

Goal

Day														
1														
2														
3														
4														
5														
6														
7														

Daily Habit Tracker
Small Steps Lead To Big Results

Month _______________

Year _______________

Goal

Day														
1														
2														
3														
4														
5														
6														
7														

Daily Habit Tracker

Small Steps Lead To Big Results

Month_____________

Year_____________

Goal

Day																
1																
2																
3																
4																
5																
6																
7																

Daily Habit Tracker

Small Steps Lead To Big Results

Month_______________

Year_______________

Goal

Day														
1														
2														
3														
4														
5														
6														
7														

Daily Habit Tracker

Small Steps Lead To Big Results

Month _______________

Year _______________

Goal

Day														
1														
2														
3														
4														
5														
6														
7														

Daily Habit Tracker

Small Steps Lead To Big Results

Month ______________

Year ______________

Goal

Day														
1														
2														
3														
4														
5														
6														
7														

Daily Habit Tracker

Small Steps Lead To Big Results

Month ________________

Year ________________

Goal

Day														
1														
2														
3														
4														
5														
6														
7														

Daily Habit Tracker

Small Steps Lead To Big Results

Month

Year

Goal

Day

1

2

3

4

5

6

7

Daily Habit Tracker
Small Steps Lead To Big Results

Month

Year

Goal

Day																
1																
2																
3																
4																
5																
6																
7																

Daily Habit Tracker

Small Steps Lead To Big Results

Month ____________

Year ____________

Goal

Day															
1															
2															
3															
4															
5															
6															
7															

Daily Habit Tracker
Small Steps Lead To Big Results

Month_____________

Year_____________

Goal

Day														
1														
2														
3														
4														
5														
6														
7														

Daily Habit Tracker

Small Steps Lead To Big Results

Month______________

Year______________

Goal

Day

1

2

3

4

5

6

7

Daily Habit Tracker

Small Steps Lead To Big Results

Month _______________

Year _______________

Goal

Day														
1														
2														
3														
4														
5														
6														
7														

Daily Habit Tracker

Small Steps Lead To Big Results

Month ___________

Year ___________

Goal

Day														
1														
2														
3														
4														
5														
6														
7														

Daily Habit Tracker

Small Steps Lead To Big Results

Month ______________

Year ______________

Goal

Day															
1															
2															
3															
4															
5															
6															
7															

Daily Habit Tracker

Small Steps Lead To Big Results

Month ___________

Year ___________

Goal

Day														
1														
2														
3														
4														
5														
6														
7														

Daily Habit Tracker

Small Steps Lead To Big Results

Month

Year

Goal

Day															
1															
2															
3															
4															
5															
6															
7															

Daily Habit Tracker
Small Steps Lead To Big Results

Month ___________

Year ___________

Goal

Day															
1															
2															
3															
4															
5															
6															
7															

Daily Habit Tracker

Small Steps Lead To Big Results

Month

Year

Goal

Day															
1															
2															
3															
4															
5															
6															
7															

Daily Habit Tracker

Small Steps Lead To Big Results

Month _______________

Year _______________

Goal

Day
1
2
3
4
5
6
7

Daily Habit Tracker

Small Steps Lead To Big Results

Month ______________

Year ______________

Goal

Day															
1															
2															
3															
4															
5															
6															
7															

Daily Habit Tracker

Small Steps Lead To Big Results

Goal

Month

Year

Day																
1																
2																
3																
4																
5																
6																
7																

Daily Habit Tracker

Small Steps Lead To Big Results

Month______________

Year______________

Goal

Day															
1															
2															
3															
4															
5															
6															
7															

Daily Habit Tracker

Small Steps Lead To Big Results

Month_______________

Year_______________

Goal

Day														
1														
2														
3														
4														
5														
6														
7														

Daily Habit Tracker

Small Steps Lead To Big Results

Month ___________

Year ___________

Goal

Day														
1														
2														
3														
4														
5														
6														
7														

Daily Habit Tracker

Small Steps Lead To Big Results

Month _______________

Year _______________

Goal

Day														
1														
2														
3														
4														
5														
6														
7														

Daily Habit Tracker

Small Steps Lead To Big Results

Month__________

Year__________

Goal

Day															
1															
2															
3															
4															
5															
6															
7															

Daily Habit Tracker

Small Steps Lead To Big Results

Month ______________

Year ______________

Goal

Day														
1														
2														
3														
4														
5														
6														
7														

Daily Habit Tracker

Small Steps Lead To Big Results

Month ___________

Year ___________

Goal

Day														
1														
2														
3														
4														
5														
6														
7														

Daily Habit Tracker

Small Steps Lead To Big Results

Month

Year

Goal

Day
1
2
3
4
5
6
7

Daily Habit Tracker

Small Steps Lead To Big Results

Month _______________

Year _______________

Goal

Day															
1															
2															
3															
4															
5															
6															
7															

Daily Habit Tracker

Small Steps Lead To Big Results

Month ______________

Year ______________

Goal

Day														
1														
2														
3														
4														
5														
6														
7														

Daily Habit Tracker

Small Steps Lead To Big Results

Month ________________

Year ________________

Goal

Day															
1															
2															
3															
4															
5															
6															
7															

Daily Habit Tracker

Small Steps Lead To Big Results

Month ______________

Year ______________

Goal

Day														
1														
2														
3														
4														
5														
6														
7														

Daily Habit Tracker

Small Steps Lead To Big Results

Month _______________

Year _______________

Goal

Day														
1														
2														
3														
4														
5														
6														
7														

Daily Habit Tracker

Small Steps Lead To Big Results

Month ________________

Year ________________

Goal

Day														
1														
2														
3														
4														
5														
6														
7														

Daily Habit Tracker
Small Steps Lead To Big Results

Month ______________

Year ______________

Goal

Day															
1															
2															
3															
4															
5															
6															
7															

Daily Habit Tracker

Small Steps Lead To Big Results

Month ______________

Year ______________

Goal

Day															
1															
2															
3															
4															
5															
6															
7															

Daily Habit Tracker

Small Steps Lead To Big Results

Month________________

Year________________

Goal

Day														
1														
2														
3														
4														
5														
6														
7														

Daily Habit Tracker

Small Steps Lead To Big Results

Month ___________

Year ___________

Goal

Day														
1														
2														
3														
4														
5														
6														
7														

Daily Habit Tracker

Small Steps Lead To Big Results

Month_______________

Year_______________

Goal

Day													
1													
2													
3													
4													
5													
6													
7													

Daily Habit Tracker

Small Steps Lead To Big Results

Month_______________

Year_______________

Goal														
Day 1														
2														
3														
4														
5														
6														
7														

Daily Habit Tracker

Small Steps Lead To Big Results

Month _______________

Year _______________

Goal

Day															
1															
2															
3															
4															
5															
6															
7															

Daily Habit Tracker

Small Steps Lead To Big Results

Month __________

Year __________

Goal

Day															
1															
2															
3															
4															
5															
6															
7															

Daily Habit Tracker

Small Steps Lead To Big Results

Month________________

Year________________

Goal

Day														
1														
2														
3														
4														
5														
6														
7														

Daily Habit Tracker

Small Steps Lead To Big Results

Month _______________

Year _______________

Goal

Day														
1														
2														
3														
4														
5														
6														
7														

Daily Habit Tracker

Small Steps Lead To Big Results

Month___________

Year___________

Goal

Day

1

2

3

4

5

6

7

Daily Habit Tracker

Small Steps Lead To Big Results

Month

Year

Goal

Day															
1															
2															
3															
4															
5															
6															
7															

Daily Habit Tracker

Small Steps Lead To Big Results

Month __________

Year __________

Goal

Day															
1															
2															
3															
4															
5															
6															
7															

Daily Habit Tracker

Small Steps Lead To Big Results

Month ________________

Year ________________

Goal

Day															
1															
2															
3															
4															
5															
6															
7															

Daily Habit Tracker

Small Steps Lead To Big Results

Month ___________

Year ___________

Goal

Day															
1															
2															
3															
4															
5															
6															
7															

Daily Habit Tracker

Small Steps Lead To Big Results

Month

Year

Goal

Day

1

2

3

4

5

6

7

Daily Habit Tracker

Small Steps Lead To Big Results

Month _______________

Year _______________

Goal

Day

1

2

3

4

5

6

7

Daily Habit Tracker

Small Steps Lead To Big Results

Month___________

Year___________

Goal

Day														
1														
2														
3														
4														
5														
6														
7														

Daily Habit Tracker
Small Steps Lead To Big Results

Month ___________

Year ___________

Goal

Day														
1														
2														
3														
4														
5														
6														
7														

Daily Habit Tracker

Small Steps Lead To Big Results

Month __________

Year __________

Goal

Day															
1															
2															
3															
4															
5															
6															
7															

Daily Habit Tracker

Small Steps Lead To Big Results

Month________

Year________

Goal

Day															
1															
2															
3															
4															
5															
6															
7															

Daily Habit Tracker

Small Steps Lead To Big Results

Month____________________

Year____________________

Goal

Day															
1															
2															
3															
4															
5															
6															
7															

Daily Habit Tracker

Small Steps Lead To Big Results

Goal

Month_____________

Year_____________

Day														
1														
2														
3														
4														
5														
6														
7														

Daily Habit Tracker

Small Steps Lead To Big Results

Month ___________

Year ___________

Goal

Day														
1														
2														
3														
4														
5														
6														
7														

Daily Habit Tracker
Small Steps Lead To Big Results

Month_____________

Year_____________

Goal

Day															
1															
2															
3															
4															
5															
6															
7															

Daily Habit Tracker

Small Steps Lead To Big Results

Month _______________

Year _______________

Goal

Day															
1															
2															
3															
4															
5															
6															
7															

Daily Habit Tracker

Small Steps Lead To Big Results

Month ___________

Year ___________

Goal

Day														
1														
2														
3														
4														
5														
6														
7														

Daily Habit Tracker

Small Steps Lead To Big Results

Month _______________

Year _______________

Goal																
Day 1																
2																
3																
4																
5																
6																
7																

Daily Habit Tracker
Small Steps Lead To Big Results

Month_______________

Year_______________

Goal

Day															
1															
2															
3															
4															
5															
6															
7															

Daily Habit Tracker

Small Steps Lead To Big Results

Month_______________

Year_______________

Goal

Day														
1														
2														
3														
4														
5														
6														
7														

Daily Habit Tracker

Small Steps Lead To Big Results

Month_____________

Year_____________

Goal

Day														
1														
2														
3														
4														
5														
6														
7														

Daily Habit Tracker

Small Steps Lead To Big Results

Month_____________

Year_____________

Goal

Day														
1														
2														
3														
4														
5														
6														
7														

Daily Habit Tracker

Small Steps Lead To Big Results

Month_______________

Year_______________

Goal

Day

1

2

3

4

5

6

7

Daily Habit Tracker

Small Steps Lead To Big Results

Month __________

Year __________

Goal

Day														
1														
2														
3														
4														
5														
6														
7														

Daily Habit Tracker

Small Steps Lead To Big Results

Month ___________

Year ___________

Goal

Day															
1															
2															
3															
4															
5															
6															
7															

Daily Habit Tracker

Small Steps Lead To Big Results

Month

Year

Goal

Day														
1														
2														
3														
4														
5														
6														
7														

Daily Habit Tracker

Small Steps Lead To Big Results

Month________________

Year_________________

Goal

Day													
1													
2													
3													
4													
5													
6													
7													

Daily Habit Tracker

Small Steps Lead To Big Results

Month________________

Year________________

Goal

Day														
1														
2														
3														
4														
5														
6														
7														

Daily Habit Tracker
Small Steps Lead To Big Results

Month ______________

Year ______________

Goal

Day														
1														
2														
3														
4														
5														
6														
7														

Daily Habit Tracker

Small Steps Lead To Big Results

Month____________

Year____________

Goal

Day														
1														
2														
3														
4														
5														
6														
7														

Daily Habit Tracker

Small Steps Lead To Big Results

Month ________

Year ________

Goal

Day															
1															
2															
3															
4															
5															
6															
7															

Daily Habit Tracker

Small Steps Lead To Big Results

Month _______________

Year _______________

Goal

Day															
1															
2															
3															
4															
5															
6															
7															

Daily Habit Tracker

Small Steps Lead To Big Results

Month ___________

Year ___________

Goal

Day														
1														
2														
3														
4														
5														
6														
7														

Daily Habit Tracker

Small Steps Lead To Big Results

Month______________

Year______________

Goal

Day															
1															
2															
3															
4															
5															
6															
7															

Daily Habit Tracker

Small Steps Lead To Big Results

Month ________________

Year ________________

Goal

Day														
1														
2														
3														
4														
5														
6														
7														

Daily Habit Tracker

Small Steps Lead To Big Results

Month ______________

Year ______________

Goal

Day															
1															
2															
3															
4															
5															
6															
7															

Daily Habit Tracker

Small Steps Lead To Big Results

Month_______________

Year_______________

Goal

Day														
1														
2														
3														
4														
5														
6														
7														

Daily Habit Tracker

Small Steps Lead To Big Results

Month_______________

Year_______________

Goal

Day														
1														
2														
3														
4														
5														
6														
7														

Daily Habit Tracker
Small Steps Lead To Big Results

Month _______________

Year _______________

Goal

Day															
1															
2															
3															
4															
5															
6															
7															

Daily Habit Tracker

Small Steps Lead To Big Results

Month ________

Year ________

Goal

Day														
1														
2														
3														
4														
5														
6														
7														

Daily Habit Tracker
Small Steps Lead To Big Results

Month ___________

Year ___________

Goal

Day															
1															
2															
3															
4															
5															
6															
7															

Daily Habit Tracker

Small Steps Lead To Big Results

Month ____________

Year ____________

Day														
1														
2														
3														
4														
5														
6														
7														

Daily Habit Tracker

Small Steps Lead To Big Results

Month

Year

Goal

Day															
1															
2															
3															
4															
5															
6															
7															

Daily Habit Tracker
Small Steps Lead To Big Results

Month

Year

Goal

Day															
1															
2															
3															
4															
5															
6															
7															

Daily Habit Tracker

Small Steps Lead To Big Results

Month___________

Year___________

Goal

Day															
1															
2															
3															
4															
5															
6															
7															

Daily Habit Tracker

Small Steps Lead To Big Results

Month_______________

Year_______________

Goal

Day															
1															
2															
3															
4															
5															
6															
7															

Daily Habit Tracker
Small Steps Lead To Big Results

Month __________

Year __________

Goal

Day														
1														
2														
3														
4														
5														
6														
7														

Daily Habit Tracker

Small Steps Lead To Big Results

Month ______________

Year ______________

Goal

Day														
1														
2														
3														
4														
5														
6														
7														

Daily Habit Tracker
Small Steps Lead To Big Results

Month _______________

Year _______________

Goal

Day															
1															
2															
3															
4															
5															
6															
7															

Daily Habit Tracker

Small Steps Lead To Big Results

Month __________

Year __________

Goal

Day													
1													
2													
3													
4													
5													
6													
7													

Daily Habit Tracker

Small Steps Lead To Big Results

Month______________

Year______________

Goal

Day															
1															
2															
3															
4															
5															
6															
7															

Daily Habit Tracker

Small Steps Lead To Big Results

Goal

Month ___________

Year ___________

Day																
1																
2																
3																
4																
5																
6																
7																

Daily Habit Tracker

Small Steps Lead To Big Results

Month ______________

Year ______________

Goal

Day															
1															
2															
3															
4															
5															
6															
7															

Daily Habit Tracker

Small Steps Lead To Big Results

Month __________

Year __________

Goal

Day

1

2

3

4

5

6

7

Daily Habit Tracker

Small Steps Lead To Big Results

Month___________

Year___________

Goal

Day														
1														
2														
3														
4														
5														
6														
7														

Daily Habit Tracker

Small Steps Lead To Big Results

Goal

Month ______________

Year ______________

Day															
1															
2															
3															
4															
5															
6															
7															

Daily Habit Tracker

Small Steps Lead To Big Results

Month ______________

Year ______________

Goal

Day															
1															
2															
3															
4															
5															
6															
7															

Daily Habit Tracker

Small Steps Lead To Big Results

Month__________

Year__________

Goal

Day															
1															
2															
3															
4															
5															
6															
7															

Daily Habit Tracker

Small Steps Lead To Big Results

Month ______________________

Year ______________________

Goal

Day														
1														
2														
3														
4														
5														
6														
7														

Daily Habit Tracker

Small Steps Lead To Big Results

Month ___________

Year ___________

Goal

Day														
1														
2														
3														
4														
5														
6														
7														

Daily Habit Tracker

Small Steps Lead To Big Results

Month ______________

Year ______________

Goal

Day															
1															
2															
3															
4															
5															
6															
7															

Daily Habit Tracker

Small Steps Lead To Big Results

Goal

Month ______________

Year ______________

Day													
1													
2													
3													
4													
5													
6													
7													

Daily Habit Tracker

Small Steps Lead To Big Results

Month

Year

Goal

Day

1

2

3

4

5

6

7

Daily Habit Tracker

Small Steps Lead To Big Results

Month_______________

Year_______________

Goal

Day														
1														
2														
3														
4														
5														
6														
7														

Daily Habit Tracker

Small Steps Lead To Big Results

Month _______________

Year _______________

Goal

Day														
1														
2														
3														
4														
5														
6														
7														

Daily Habit Tracker

Small Steps Lead To Big Results

Month ___________

Year ___________

Goal

Day														
1														
2														
3														
4														
5														
6														
7														

Daily Habit Tracker

Small Steps Lead To Big Results

Month_______________

Year_______________

Goal

Day														
1														
2														
3														
4														
5														
6														
7														

Daily Habit Tracker

Small Steps Lead To Big Results

Month ___________

Year ___________

Goal

Day														
1														
2														
3														
4														
5														
6														
7														

Daily Habit Tracker

Small Steps Lead To Big Results

Month ___________

Year ___________

Goal

Day														
1														
2														
3														
4														
5														
6														
7														

Daily Habit Tracker

Small Steps Lead To Big Results

Month ________________

Year ________________

Goal

Day															
1															
2															
3															
4															
5															
6															
7															

Daily Habit Tracker

Small Steps Lead To Big Results

Month ______________

Year ______________

Goal

Day															
1															
2															
3															
4															
5															
6															
7															

Daily Habit Tracker

Small Steps Lead To Big Results

Month________________

Year________________

Goal

Day															
1															
2															
3															
4															
5															
6															
7															

Daily Habit Tracker

Small Steps Lead To Big Results

Month_______________

Year_______________

Goal

Day															
1															
2															
3															
4															
5															
6															
7															

Daily Habit Tracker

Small Steps Lead To Big Results

Month _______________

Year _______________

Goal

Day														
1														
2														
3														
4														
5														
6														
7														

Daily Habit Tracker

Small Steps Lead To Big Results

Month__________

Year__________

Goal

Day

1

2

3

4

5

6

7

Daily Habit Tracker

Small Steps Lead To Big Results

Month_______________

Year_______________

Goal

Day														
1														
2														
3														
4														
5														
6														
7														

Daily Habit Tracker

Small Steps Lead To Big Results

Month ______________

Year ______________

Goal

Day															
1															
2															
3															
4															
5															
6															
7															

Daily Habit Tracker

Small Steps Lead To Big Results

Month________________

Year________________

Goal

Day														
1														
2														
3														
4														
5														
6														
7														

Daily Habit Tracker
Small Steps Lead To Big Results

Month________________

Year________________

Goal

Day														
1														
2														
3														
4														
5														
6														
7														

Daily Habit Tracker

Small Steps Lead To Big Results

Month _______________

Year _______________

Goal

Day													
1													
2													
3													
4													
5													
6													
7													

Daily Habit Tracker

Small Steps Lead To Big Results

Month_______________

Year_______________

Goal

Day															
1															
2															
3															
4															
5															
6															
7															

Daily Habit Tracker

Small Steps Lead To Big Results

Month

Year

Goal

Day

1

2

3

4

5

6

7

Daily Habit Tracker

Small Steps Lead To Big Results

Month ___________

Year ___________

Goal

Day														
1														
2														
3														
4														
5														
6														
7														

Daily Habit Tracker

Small Steps Lead To Big Results

Month _______________

Year _______________

Goal

Day														
1														
2														
3														
4														
5														
6														
7														

Daily Habit Tracker

Small Steps Lead To Big Results

Month ______________

Year ______________

Goal

Day														
1														
2														
3														
4														
5														
6														
7														

Daily Habit Tracker

Small Steps Lead To Big Results

Month ___________

Year ___________

Goal

Day														
1														
2														
3														
4														
5														
6														
7														

Daily Habit Tracker

Small Steps Lead To Big Results

Month __________

Year __________

Goal

Day														
1														
2														
3														
4														
5														
6														
7														

Daily Habit Tracker
Small Steps Lead To Big Results

Month_______________

Year_______________

Goal

Day														
1														
2														
3														
4														
5														
6														
7														

Daily Habit Tracker

Small Steps Lead To Big Results

Month ______________

Year ______________

Goal

Day															
1															
2															
3															
4															
5															
6															
7															

Daily Habit Tracker

Small Steps Lead To Big Results

Month

Year

Goal

Day

1

2

3

4

5

6

7

Daily Habit Tracker

Small Steps Lead To Big Results

Month_______________

Year_______________

Goal

Day															
1															
2															
3															
4															
5															
6															
7															

Daily Habit Tracker

Small Steps Lead To Big Results

Month_____________

Year_____________

Goal

Day															
1															
2															
3															
4															
5															
6															
7															

Daily Habit Tracker

Small Steps Lead To Big Results

Month _______________

Year _______________

Goal

Day													
1													
2													
3													
4													
5													
6													
7													

Daily Habit Tracker

Small Steps Lead To Big Results

Month___________

Year___________

Goal

Day
1
2
3
4
5
6
7

Daily Habit Tracker

Small Steps Lead To Big Results

Month ___________

Year ___________

Goal

Day														
1														
2														
3														
4														
5														
6														
7														

Daily Habit Tracker

Small Steps Lead To Big Results

Month____________

Year____________

Goal

Day													
1													
2													
3													
4													
5													
6													
7													

Daily Habit Tracker

Small Steps Lead To Big Results

Month_______________

Year_______________

Goal

Day														
1														
2														
3														
4														
5														
6														
7														

Daily Habit Tracker

Small Steps Lead To Big Results

Month ________

Year ________

Goal

Day														
1														
2														
3														
4														
5														
6														
7